Contents

Preface

A Clinical Guide to Pediatric Infectious Disease arose from ten years of lectures to medical students, residents, and community-based attending physicians. The need was there for a text that would provide a straightforward laboratory and clinical approach to the numerous infectious diseases encountered by physicians who care for children. The evaluation and treatment of infections comprises a significant part of any pediatric practice. General practitioners too are often required to provide evaluations of patients with specialized conditions such as fever, neutropenia, and infection following organ transplantation.

This book is intended to give both the trainee and general practitioner a quick reference, supplying answers to the fundamental questions of "which bacteria?" "what do I order?" and "how long do I treat?" that frequently arise in a busy office practice or hospital ward. Also included are basic concepts such as the use of a gram stain, interpretation of bacterial cultures, and the meaning of a minimal inhibital concentration—fundamental issues for infectious disease specialists.

This text is not meant to replace other more extensive volumes available on the subject; rather, it is meant to serve as an introduction to a clinical approach that can be utilized when facing the classic infectious diseases of pediatrics.

This book is dedicated to my parents (Michael and Barbara)
and my first teachers, Parvin Azimi, M.D.
and Ann Petru M.D.
It could not have been written without them.

Acknowledgments

This project could not have happened without the help of some very special people. The author wishes to thank Department Chair John Mace, M.D. and Lippincott Williams & Wilkins Acquisitions Editor Timothy Hiscock for their initial enthusiasm for the project. Anne Sydor and Louise Bierig lent their considerable patience and editing expertise to the preparation of the manuscript. Finally, great appreciation is expressed to Ann Elliott and Beatrice Strayer for their help with the endless revisions of the manuscript.

1

Laboratory Diagnosis of Pediatric Infectious Disease

A variety of laboratory tests are used in pediatric infectious disease. Useful techniques include blood cultures, Gram stain, serology, and determination of minimal inhibitory concentration (MIC). This chapter discusses these methods and addresses the most common questions regarding the interpretation of these tests.

Interpretation of a Positive Culture

Clinicians are often required to determine whether a bacterial culture is "real," that is, represents a true invasive bacterial infection. The accurate interpretation of a positive bacterial culture requires an understanding of **colonization**, **contamination**, and **invasive infection**.

DISTINGUISHING COLONIZATION, CONTAMINATION, AND INVASIVE INFECTIONS

Definitions

Colonization refers to the isolation of bacteria or fungi from an area of the body that is not expected to be sterile, including skin surfaces and tracheostomy tubes. These surfaces are in contact with the outside environment, and the presence of bacteria is not indicative of invasive disease. Within hours after birth, neonates become colonized with a variety of bacteria and even fungal pathogens. Cultures of their nose, mouth, or skin would be positive for numerous bacteria and yeast. Usually, organisms residing in these areas do so without ill effects to the host.

Contamination refers to the presence of an organism isolated from a site expected to be sterile. These organisms are not causing disease; rather, their isolation is the result of a break in sterile technique during sampling. Contaminated body fluids can include blood, peritoneal fluid, and even cerebrospinal fluid.

Invasive infection refers to the presence of bacteria and fungi that are causing clinical disease.

Colonization versus Invasive Infection

In evaluating a positive culture from a nonsterile area, the first issue is whether the culture represents colonization or true infection. This is typically an assessment required with a skin or endotracheal tube culture. One must rely on the **overall clinical picture** of the patient. A skin culture obtained in the context of cellulitis or obvious wound infection would likely represent a true infection. A positive skin culture obtained on intact or normal-looking skin usually represents colonization.

In evaluating an endotracheal tube culture, it is also important to consider the entire clinical picture. Many studies have evaluated the optimal method for determining whether an endotracheal tube or tracheostomy tube culture represents a ventilator-associated pneumonia (invasive disease) or routine colonization. Generally, a clinical decision is made involving an evaluation of the patient's vital signs, respiratory status, oxygenation, and chest x-ray. An endotracheal tube culture obtained in a stable patient without respiratory deterioration is often deemed colonization. A positive endotracheal tube culture taken in the setting of decreasing oxygenation, an increase in ventilatory status, fever, leukocytosis, or new pulmonary infiltrates would likely represent a true invasive pathogen.

Contaminant versus Invasive Infection

The second exercise frequently facing the clinician is determining whether an isolate from a sterile body site (such as blood or cerebrospinal fluid) is a contaminant or a true infection. The following case provides an example of the importance of making an accurate determination.

A term newborn with a history of intrauterine drug exposure was evaluated for a low-grade fever. A blood culture was obtained and grew *Staphylococcus aureus*. Repeat blood cultures were negative, and this isolate was thought to be a contami-

---

"Always"

Group A streptococcus (*Streptococcus pyogenes*)
Group B streptococcus (*Streptococcus agalactiae*)
Streptococcus pneumoniae
Gram-negative rods
Fungi
Staphylococcus aureus
Neisseria meningitis

"Sometimes"

Coagulase-negative staphylococcus (*Staphylococcus epidermidis*)
Corynebacterium species
Bacillus species

---

nant. Over the next 2 weeks, the child became increasing irritable; this was attributed to drug withdrawal. Phenobarbital was given with little effect. After 2 weeks, the infant's knee joint became swollen and ultimately ruptured, discharging purulent fluid. Culture of this fluid grew *S. aureus*.

This story stresses the importance of an accurate determination of whether a positive blood culture constitutes a true infection. Although the bacteremia itself may be transient, the bacteria may come to rest at secondary sites such as the brain or bone. Therefore, it is wise to treat aggressively all pathogens that are thought to be "real," even if repeat blood cultures are negative. Infection at secondary sites, left untreated, can cause major morbidity and even mortality.

A good system to use is the "always/sometimes" system. Certain pathogens, when isolated from a sterile site (such as blood), are always considered true infections and require treatment. These pathogens should not readily be considered contaminants.

A good system to use is the "always/sometimes" system. Certain pathogens, when isolated from a sterile site (such as blood), are always considered true infections and require treatment. These pathogens should not readily be considered contaminants.

There are some bacteria that, when isolated in blood or spinal fluid, can be either invasive pathogens or contaminants. Often, these organisms reside on skin surfaces, facilitating the contamination in cultures. These can be referred to as the "sometimes" pathogens. Despite these organisms often being contaminants, care must be taken in making this designation. Generally speaking, the more immunocompromised a patient (particularly in the setting of indwelling catheters), the greater the chance of skin flora becoming a true invasive pathogen.

As in the evaluation of a skin or endotracheal tube culture, a clinical context is needed. A well patient with a single positive blood culture for coagulase-negative staphylococcus usually warrants no therapy. A febrile oncology patient with an indwelling catheter and a blood culture for *Corynebacterium* or *Bacillus* species should be strongly considered for treatment because these organisms represent pathogens in this patient population.

Quantitation of bacterial colonies is an additional technique considered helpful in interpretation of blood cultures. Peripheral cultures that grow more than 50 colony forming units (CFUs) likely represent infection, whereas peripheral blood cultures with less than 5 CFUs usually represents contamination. Unfortunately, the ability to perform quantitative culture is often not available.

GRAM-STAIN MORPHOLOGY

The Gram stain is often the first laboratory test returned to a clinician caring for an ill child, usually reported as an organism growing in blood or cerebrospinal fluid. Correct interpretation of a positive Gram stain in the blood or cerebrospinal fluid can

---

Gram Stain Game

The Gram stain divides bacteria into two groups. Gram-positive bacteria retain crystal violet stain, whereas gram-negative bacteria do not and appear red. Gram stains are also designated in terms of morphology and configuration; bacteria are typically designated as cocci, rods, clusters, and chains (Table 1.1).

TABLE 1.1. *Gram Stain Game*

Gram-positive cocci in clusters
   Staphylococcus aureus (coagulase positive)
   Methicillin-resistant staphylococci
   Coagulase-negative staphylococci (coagulase negative)
Gram-positive cocci in chains
   Streptococcus pyogenes (group A streptococci)
   Streptococcus agalactiae (group B streptococci)
   Viridans streptococcus
   Enterococcus species
   Streptococcus pneumoniae
Gram-positive rods
   Acid fast:
     Mycobacteria
     Nocardia species
     Rhodococcus species
   Non-acid fast
     Corynebacterium species
     Bacillus anthrax, Bacillus cereus
     Listeria monocytogenes
Gram-negative rods
   Community acquired
     Escherichia coli
     Haemophilus influenzae
     Salmonella species
   Hospital acquired
     Pseudomonas species
     Enterobacter species
     Serratia species
Gram-negative diplococci
   Neisseria meningitidis
   Moraxella catarrhalis

---

lead to optimal antibiotic management, which in turn can have a significant effect on patient outcome. One way to approach the correct interpretation of a Gram stain is the "Gram stain game". This can be done by dividing the isolate into major categories based on Gram stain morphology. The possible isolates with a given Gram stain morphology can then be evaluated in regard to the particular patient.

Gram-positive Cocci in Clusters

Clusters of gram-positive cocci usually represent *Staphylococcus* species infection. Staphylococci are divided traditionally into two groups based on the coagulase test. *S. aureus* is the most common coagulase-positive isolate. Coagulase-negative staphylococci include more than 30 species, the most common of which is *Staphylococcus epidermidis*. *S. epidermidis* is a common infection of surgical catheters and implanted foreign bodies and is a common contaminant found in blood cultures. Methicillin-resistant staphylococci should also be considered in the initial evaluation of any Gram stain showing gram-positive cocci in clusters. Once thought to occur primarily in hospitalized patients, a large percentage of community-acquired *S. aureus* infections are now methicillin resistant. When this Gram stain is isolated from an ill patient and empiric treatment is warranted, vancomycin provides empiric coverage.

Gram-positive Cocci in Chains

In children, chains of gram-positive cocci are usually seen in five organisms:

• Group A streptococcus
• Group B streptococcus
• *Streptococcus pneumoniae*
• Viridans streptococci
• *Enterococcus* species

These are classified in numerous ways. One of the most frequently used systems classifies the ability of the organism to lyse red blood cells on a blood agar plate. β-Hemolytic streptococci produce complete hemolysis on sheep blood agar. α-Hemolytic organisms produce partial hemolysis, resulting in a green or a grayish zone surrounding colonies. Nonhemolytic organisms impart no hemolysis on blood auger plate.

Group A streptococcus is a β-hemolytic organism that is implicated in pharyngitis as well as toxic shock syndrome.

Group B streptococcus is also β-hemolytic and is a common colonizer of the female genital tract that is a primary cause of neonatal sepsis and meningitis.

Streptococcus pneumoniae is the major cause of otitis media and bacterial pneumonia in toddlers. It is typically α-hemolytic.

Viridans streptococcus is not a single organism but rather a large number of different streptococci. These α-hemolytic streptococci reside in the gastrointestinal (GI) tract and are implicated in transient bacteremia, endocarditis, and GI-related septicemia.

***Enterococcus* species** are nonhemolytic organisms residing in the GI tract that is often implicated in endocarditis and septicemia secondary to abdominal trauma.

Clinical context can help the clinician make the best guess as to the offending pathogen. A neonate who is clinically septic and has a blood culture isolate of gram-positive cocci in chains is likely to have group B streptococcus; less likely are viridans streptococci and enterococci. Empiric treatment with ampicillin and gentamicin covers these pathogens best. A toddler with a diagnosis of bacterial meningitis and gram-positive cocci in chains seen in the cerebrospinal fluid is likely to have *Streptococcus pneumoniae*. In this case, the best empiric treatment is vancomycin plus a third-generation cephalosporin. A patient who has intraabdominal sepsis with gram-positive cocci in chains isolated from nonblood or peritoneal culture is likely to have viridans streptococci or enterococci because these organisms reside in the GI tract. In this case, ampicillin with gentamicin or vancomycin provides good coverage.

Gram-positive Rods

The gram-positive rods are an unusual group of pathogens that can cause disease in specialized conditions. In evaluating this group, a helpful first step is to determine whether the organism is acid-fast positive.

Gram-positive rods that are acid-fast positive include the following:

- Mycobacteria
- *Nocardia* species
- *Rhodococcus* species

Gram-positive rods that are not acid-fast positive include the following:

- *Listeria monocytogenes*
- *Bacillus* species
- *Corynebacterium* species
- *Clostridium* species

Rhodococcus (formally *Corynebacterium*) ***equi*** is a gram-positive rod that may be partially acid fast. Primarily an animal pathogen, it has become recognized as a human pathogen that causes respiratory disease and sepsis in immunocompromised hosts. The organism may cause a necrotizing pneumonia associated with bacteremia that can resemble *Mycobacterium tuberculosis* or *Nocardia* species infection. These bacteria are resistant to β-lactam antibiotics and often require prolonged treatment with vancomycin.

Nocardia **species** are weakly acid fast. In immunocompromised patients, including those with chronic granulomatous disease and those receiving long-term corticosteroid treatment, chronic pneumonia may be seen. Pulmonary disease with dissemination to skin and brain is frequently encountered. *Nocardia* pneumonia often appears as a consolidation process resembling mycobacterial disease. Long-term treatment with trimethoprim-sulfamethoxazole is usually needed.

Listeria monocytogenes affects neonates and immunocompromised patients. Neonates have early-onset and late-onset syndromes similar to group B streptococcal infection. *Listeria* is an aerobic, non-spore-forming, motile gram-positive rod that is usually easily identified by the laboratory once the initial morphology of gram-positive rod is confirmed. Antibiotic therapy includes the combination treatment of ampicillin and gentamicin.

Bacillus **species** are non-acid-fast gram-positive rods. The major member of this species in terms of past and present historical importance remains *Bacillus anthracis*. Anthrax is caused when spores are inhaled, digested, or come in close contact with body surfaces. Skin infections begin as painless lesions around which vesicles develop. The vesicles then progress to an eschar and are often accompanied by marked edema. Inhalation anthrax begins with flulike illness which progresses to respiratory failure, sepsis, and meningitis. Although anthrax remains rare, it should be considered in the proper epidemiologic and clinical contexts.

The other major *Bacillus* species is *Bacillus cereus*, an endotoxin-producing spore. This organism can cause endophthalmitis and neonatal sepsis. A gram-positive rod isolated from a septic neonate, even if the lab indicates it is not *Listeria* species, should not automatically be considered a contaminant. *B. cereus* is resistant to β-lactam antibiotics and requires vancomycin for treatment.

Corynebacterium **species** are commonly referred to as *diphtheroids* and are non-motile, non-acid-fast organisms that are the most common gram-positive rod species isolated in blood cultures. Corynebacteria are common in the environment and are part of the normal skin flora. Although frequently the cause of contamination in blood cultures, their isolation can also signify the presence of true invasive disease. *Corynebacterium diphtheriae*, the cause of diphtheria, is rare in developed countries. *Corynebacterium jeikeium*, previously known as *Corynebacterium* group JK, is an opportunistic pathogen increasingly seen in hematology and oncology patients. *Corynebacterium striatum* is reported as a cause of serious infection in the immunocompromised host. Patients with leukopenia and indwelling catheters are also particularly susceptible. *C. jeikeium* is resistant to most antibiotics and requires vancomycin for treatment. Specific identification of an organism labeled diphtheroid or corynebacteria should be strongly considered if the patient is immunosuppressed or seriously ill.

Clostridium **species** are anaerobic bacilli that reside in the GI tract and the environment. These bacteria usually require anaerobic media to grow. These organisms often secrete toxins that are involved in the pathogenesis of the disease process.

These include *Clostridium perfringens* (gas gangrene), *Clostridium botulinum* (associated with paralysis), *Clostridium difficile* (antibiotic-associated diarrhea), and *Clostridium tetani* (tetanus).

Gram-negative Rods

It is helpful to divide the gram-negative rods into two basic groups: those that are community acquired and those causing nosocomial infections.

The community-acquired gram-negative rods include the following:

- *Escherichia coli*
- *Haemophilus influenzae*
- *Salmonella* species

The incidence of haemophilus type B disease has greatly diminished since the introduction of the conjugate vaccine. After the newborn period (when *E. coli* predominates), a toddler with fever, gastroenteritis, and gram-negative rods in the blood is likely to have a *Salmonella* species infection. A third-generation cephalosporin in these instances is usually adequate.

The nosocomial gram-negative rods are a different group of organisms that includes the following:

- *Klebsiella* species
- *Enterobacter* species
- *Serratia* species

These organisms are noteworthy for their rapid induction of β-lactamase production. Even if they are initially sensitive to semisynthetic penicillins or cephalosporins, within a few days, these organisms can become resistant.

β-Lactam Sensitivity Cannot Be Assumed

Never rely on a third-generation cephalosporin alone when faced with a gram-negative sepsis in a severely ill patient in a hospital or intensive care setting. Empiric treatment with more broad-spectrum coverage (such as amikacin, imipenem, or a fluoroquinolone) should be considered until final identification and sensitivities are known. Numerous studies point to the significance of the early correct treatment of nosocomial gram-negative infection on overall morbidity and mortality.

Extended-Spectrum β-Lactamase (ESBL)

In addition to empiric treatment for infection with presumed β-lactamase-producing organisms, understanding the correct laboratory diagnosis of these pathogens is critical.

Various organisms, typically gram-negative bacteria, can produce extended-spectrum β-lactamase (ESBL) by a variety of means. These β-lactamases are often secondary to encoded plasmids and cause structural changes in the β-lactamase protein that can increase its activity to include the third- and fourth-generation cephalosporins and most semisynthetic penicillins. Patients most likely to develop these ESBL-producing organisms are those with prolonged hospitalization or multiple courses of broad-spectrum antibiotics.

The initial clinical suspicion for ESBL begins with evaluation of the antibiotic resistance panel of an isolated organism. ESBL-producing organisms typically have reduced susceptibility to all cephalosporins and semisynthetic penicillins. The National Committee for Clinical Laboratory Standards (NCCLS) has proposed screening criteria for ESBL production; an MIC greater than 4 μg/mL for ceftdzidime is thought to be particularly worrisome. Confirmatory testing involves "double-disk" Kirby-Bauer methodology. Zones of inhibition around an isolate are measured against disks of third-generation cephalosporins alone and then in combination with disks containing the β-lactamase inhibitor clavulanic acid. A more than 5-mm increase in the zone of inhibition when the disks are combined usually indicates ESBL production. If the laboratory does confirm an ESBL-producing strain, β-lactam antibiotics such as semisynthetic penicillins or cephalosporins should not be used, regardless of *in vitro* antibiotic reporting. Most authorities suggest carbapenems (imipenem) as front-line therapy for ESBL-producing organisms.

Gram-negative Diplococci

Two major organisms are in the group of gram-negative diplococci, the most important being *Neisseria meningitidis*. *N. meningitidis* remains a major cause of overwhelming sepsis and meningitis. *Moraxella catarrhalis* is a common cause of lower respiratory infection and otitis media in children; it occasionally can cause invasive bacteremic disease. *Neisseria* species remain susceptible to penicillin, whereas *Moraxella* species have a higher incidence of β-lactam production; these organisms require second- or third-generation cephalosporins.

Serologic Diagnosis in Infectious Disease

Many agents in pediatric infectious disease are difficult to culture. These include atypical bacteria, such as *Rickettsia, Legionella*, and *Chlamydia* species, and viral pathogens. The measurements of serum antibodies provide the clinician with a valuable tool in diagnosing infection.

SEROLOGIC DIAGNOSIS

Two major points regarding serologic diagnosis must be remembered when using this diagnostic technique. First is that most serology measures immunoglobulin G (IgG) antibodies that readily cross the placenta. These maternal antibodies can persist in an infant's circulation for many months and sometimes for up to a year, complicating the interpretation of these tests in young children.

The second potential pitfall is that there is a very high incidence of "background" IgG serology. Most individuals have been exposed to numerous pathogens and are positive for a variety of IgG antibodies. A patient with acute hepatitis and an IgG antibody for hepatitis A does not have proven acute hepatitis A infection. The diagnosis of acute infection often must be made by more sophisticated means. Specific IgM serology often is used because IgM represents the earliest antibody response and is often elevated in the setting of acute infection. The diagnosis of acute infection can also be made by a single IgG titer; a sufficiently high IgG titer is thought not to represent background serology and can only be present in the context of an acute infection. An additional method of diagnosing an acute or recent infection is to use paired serology to show a rise in IgG antibodies; a four-fold rise in IgG antibody titers measured several weeks apart is also taken as evidence of recent infection.

Direct Immunofluorescent Antibody

In addition to serology, other methods can be used to document the presence of difficult-to-culture organisms. Direct fluorescent antibody (DFA) staining employs the use of specific antibodies linked to a light-emitting material. The antibody binds to the infecting pathogen and can then be visualized by a specially equipped microscope to detect the emitted fluorescence. The advantage of this technique is that it can be done rapidly, often in less than 24 hours.

Minimal Inhibitory Concentration

The MIC refers to the lowest concentration of an antibiotic that visibly inhibits the *in vitro* growth of an organism. This information can help to determine whether a given antibiotic can be used for treatment of specific bacteria. There are several ways of determining the MIC.

DILUTION TESTING

Dilution testing is the major methodology in determining MIC (Fig. 1.1). An early method for dilution testing actually used rows of standard test tubes (macrodilution method). Typically, eight or more concentrations of an antibiotic were used

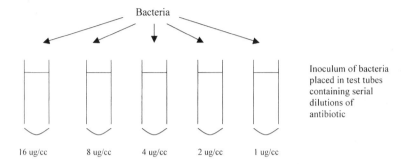

Bacteria

Inoculum of bacteria placed in test tubes containing serial dilutions of antibiotic

16 ug/cc   8 ug/cc   4 ug/cc   2 ug/cc   1 ug/cc

In 24 hours, the concentration that fails to inhibit growth in test tube results in the test tube becoming cloudy.

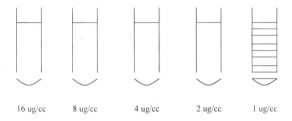

16 ug/cc   8 ug/cc   4 ug/cc   2 ug/cc   1 ug/cc

Minimal Inhibitory Concentration = 2.0 ug/cc

FIG. 1.1. Minimal inhibitory concentration (MIC).

with twofold dilutions (16, 8, 4, 2, and 1 μg/mL). A standard amount of bacteria, usually 5×10^5 CFUs/mL, is inoculated in each test tube. In 24 hours, the tubes are examined, and the first concentration in which there is no visible growth is determined to be the MIC.

Tube dilution has been modified by miniaturization techniques. Microdilution trays that contain 96 wells of 100μL each allow up to 12 antibiotics to be tested at one time. Visible growth in a specific tube dilution can be determined visually or by automated photometers.

Another method for calculating MIC is the disk diffusion method (Kirby-Bauer method), which involves a bacterial inoculation of 1 to 2×10^8 CFUs/mL to an agar plate, on which is placed an antibiotic disk. After 24 hours of incubation, diameters of the zone of inhibition around the antibiotic disks are measured to the nearest millimeter (Fig. 1.2). This zone-of-inhibition diameter is related to the susceptibility of the isolate (i.e., linear regression analysis of zone diameter plotted against log 2 MIC values). This test is attractive in that it is simple and can be performed in community hospital laboratories. However, the disadvantage of this test is that it provides only a qualitative result rather than a quantitative MIC.

Nonetheless, this diffusion method remains in place in many laboratories and can be helpful in many basic infections.

The NCCLS provides guidelines for methodology in determining MICs. It also determines the "breakpoints" (i.e., the MIC results for a given drug that are interpreted as susceptible, intermediate, or resistant). The breakpoints are made through an analysis of several factors, including data on achievable drug concentrations, the results of clinical trials, and appraisal of toxicities.

Although the MIC and breakpoints are often used in selecting a particular antibiotic, additional variables need to be considered. Drug concentrations within the patient may change over time or may not represent the actual free drug concentration at the site of infection. Drugs that are excreted renally may actually have higher concentrations in the urine; drugs that do not cross the blood-brain barrier may actually have reduced levels within the cerebrospinal fluid. Multiple additional factors, such as toxin production, individual host response, and concentration of antibiotic at the site of infection, are important and can determine response. Breakpoints often need to be reevaluated as new data emerge regarding the development of antibiotic resistance. The "90-60 rule" has been proposed; this rule states that a susceptible isolate will respond 90% of the time, whereas a resistant isolate will respond only about 60% of the time.

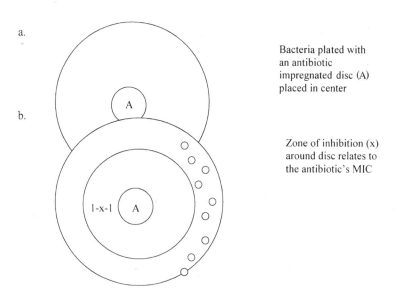

FIG. 1.2. Disc diffusion method (Kirby-Bauer).

Pharmacodynamics in Infectious Disease

In addition to MIC calculations, the advancing field of pharmacodynamics has led to additional refinement in the way clinicians use the MIC and administer antibiotics.

PHARMACODYNAMIC CLASSIFICATION

Concentration-dependent Killing

For antibiotics in this group, such as aminoglycosides and the fluoroquinolones, the rate of killing of an organism is dependent on the concentration of the antibiotic above the MIC. High ratios of peak drug concentration to MIC (10:1) are correlated with lower development of resistance and improved clinical outcome. The use of once-daily aminoglycoside dosing is based on this principle; increasing the milligram per kilogram dose given once a day increases the peak concentration and therefore increases the ratio of peak drug concentration to MIC. Additionally, the risk for nephrotoxicity with aminoglycosides is thought to be related to increased trough concentration for an extended period of time. It is possible that this could be reduced with once-daily dosing because there is an increased period of time with lower undetectable drug concentrations.

Although there has been increasing acceptance of once-daily aminoglycoside dosing in adults, it has yet to become standard practice in children. Most published data regarding the use of once-daily dosing in adults are based on a short duration of therapy. Children may have different volumes of distribution and excretion patterns than adults, leading to different outcomes. There is concern that a higher dose given once daily, often 6 mg/kg, may be associated with higher ototoxicity if used for an extended periods. Although once-daily dosing remains an attractive theory, it has not been definitively proved in pediatric studies. It is possible that once-daily dosing will gain increasing acceptance in pediatrics as clinical experience with this therapy increases.

Time-dependent Killing

This pharmacodynamic pattern is seen with β-lactam antibiotics such as penicillin, cephalosporins, and carbapenems. Maximal killing is related not to the concentration ratio above the MIC, but rather to the time above the MIC. For penicillins and cephalosporins, the plasma concentration needs to exceed the MIC for 50% to 70% of the dosing interval for maximal effectiveness. In the case of carbapenems, the plasma concentration should exceed the MIC for at least 40% of the dosing interval. It is for this reason that these drugs are often considered for continuous infusions, so that the plasma concentrations will continually be above the MIC. Like once-daily therapy for aminoglycoside administration, there is minimal clinical experience in pediatrics, and it is not used extensively in children's hospitals at this time.

The art of optimal antibiotic administration is an evolving one. MIC determinations, clinical experience, the site of infections, and pharmacodynamics will all play a role in future studies regarding antibiotic use.

SELECTED READINGS

American Academy of Pediatrics. *Report of the Committee on Infectious Disease 2003*, 26th ed.

Feigin R, Cherry J. *Textbook of pediatric infectious diseases,* 5th ed. Philadelphia: WB Saunders, 2003.

Long SS, Pickering LK, Proter CG, eds. *Principles and practice of infectious diseases*, 2nd ed. Philadelphia: Churchill Livingstone.

2

Osteomyelitis and
Septic Arthritis

Mechanisms of Infection

There are three basic mechanisms of infection: (a) direct inoculation, (b) hematogenous spread, and (c) contiguous spread from an adjacent area. The hallmark of pediatric infectious disease is infection by hematogenous spread.

ETIOLOGY

Children are colonized with a variety of bacteria; a culture of the nasopharynx of an asymptomatic child could yield any number of bacteria, including *Staphylococcus aureus* and *Streptococcus pneumoniae*. Usually, these organisms reside on body surfaces with no ill effects. However, by a process not always well defined, these colonizing bacteria enter the bloodstream.

Once the bacteria enter the bloodstream, numerous things can occur (Fig. 2.1). Bacteremia can be transient and resolve without sequelae; this is often the case with viridans streptococci. Bacteremia, by its very presence in the systemic circulation, can cause overwhelming sepsis, as is often the case with *Neisseria meningitidis*. Bacteria can also be deposited in secondary sites, such as the cerebrospinal fluid or bone.

The bones are a frequent site of secondary infection because the blood supply takes a hairpin turn at the metaphyses of long bones, increasing the chance of the bacteria being deposited. This secondary seeding of bones from the blood is the major mechanism of pediatric osteomyelitis. This is in contrast to adults, who usually acquire osteomyelitis from direct inoculation following trauma or surgical procedures.

Pyogenic arthritis develops in a fashion similar to osteomyelitis, whereby blood-borne organisms are deposited in the synovium of the joint space. Similar to the long bones of children, the joint space is highly vascularized and is an area where bacteremic organisms are readily deposited. Bacterial arthritis can also spread from a contiguous osteomyelitis; blood vessels can deposit infection from the metaphysis

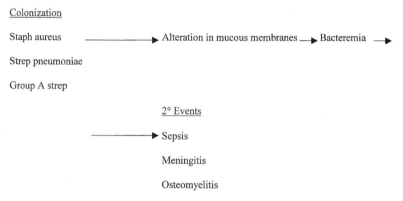

FIG. 2.1. Spread of bacteria from the bloodstream

into the joint space. The organisms of septic arthritis are similar to those of osteomyelitis. *S. aureus* is the most common organisms, followed by *S. pneumoniae, Kingella kingae,* and group A streptococcus.

PRESENTATION

The hallmark of pediatric osteomyelitis or septic arthritis is fever and localized pain. In the toddler whose verbal skills may not be sufficiently developed, the presentation may be simply fever and refusal to walk. It is for this reason that for many clinicians, fever and refusal to walk in a child indicates osteomyelitis or septic arthritis until proven otherwise. Septic arthritis of the hip is of particular concern to pediatricians because this joint space cannot be visualized directly on physical examination.

DIAGNOSIS

Clinical Clues to Diagnosis of Septic Arthritis of the Hip

The classic picture of a child with septic arthritis of the hip is a child holding the hip flexed and in external rotation. Often, the clinical picture can be subtle, with the major clinical clues being decreased leg motion and crying with diaper changes. There has been great interest in developing a clinical model for predicting that the child with fever, limp, and hip pain has either toxic synovitis or septic arthritis of the hip. One frequently quoted study indicated four major clinical variables: peripheral white blood count greater than $12,000/m^3$, sedimentation rate greater than 40 mm/h, fever, and non–weight bearing. When none of the clinical variables are present, the probability of pyogenic arthritis is less than 0.2%; the probability of septic arthritis of the hip increased to 93% and 99.6% when three and four clinical variables, respectively, are seen.

EVALUATION

When facing the clinical condition of the febrile child who is not walking, it is necessary to pursue a logical clinical and laboratory evaluation. A complete physical examination is mandatory. Point tenderness should be sought in an attempt to localize potential infected areas. A careful examination should always include full range of motion of the hips.

Rapid Diagnosis of Septic Arthritis of the Hip

Rapid diagnosis of septic arthritis of the hip is particularly important because the tight confines of the hip joint in the setting of a purulent infection can rapidly compromise the arterial blood supply. If there is any question about the existence of septic arthritis of the hip, an ultrasound of the hip should be obtained. If fluid is seen by this study, one cannot easily determine whether this fluid is purulent or secondary to a transient viral infection (toxic synovitis).

Stepwise evaluation for suspected septic hip includes the following:

1. Child with fever, refusal to walk
2. Physical examination: assess for point tenderness, hip pain, and decreased internal rotation of hip.
3. Widening of joint space suggests septic arthritis (Fig. 2.2). Plain films can rule out trauma and slipped epiphyses.
4. Laboratory evaluations: sedimentation rate, blood culture, complete blood count
5. Ultrasound of hips: rule out effusion
6. If any effusion is present, aspiration by orthopedic surgeon or interventional radiology is indicated.

All joints that appear swollen and erythematous should be aspirated with fluid sent for Gram stain, culture, and white blood cell count. If purulent fluid is present or an aspirate reveals greater than 100,000 white blood cells/m^3 or positive Gram stain, the diagnosis of septic arthritis is made.

If point tenderness is elicited, plain films of the area should be done. Changes on plain films from osteomyelitis are often not apparent for at least 14 days; the real purpose of plain films is to rule out any other reason for the clinical presentation, such as an occult fracture or foreign body. Complete blood counts, sedimentation rate, and blood cultures are also useful. Although only 50% of patients with osteomyelitis have elevations in their white blood cell count, 90% of patients with osteomyelitis or septic arthritis have elevation in the sedimentation rate or C-reactive protein. Given the mechanism of the disease in pediatric osteomyelitis, blood cultures should be obtained and are positive in up to 30% of cases.

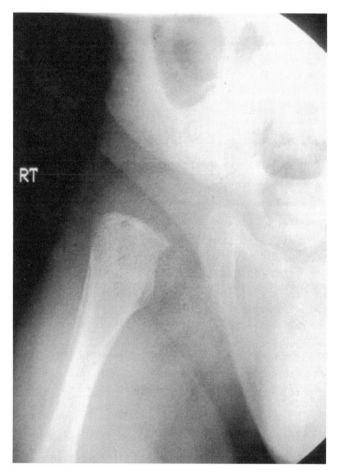

FIG. 2.2. Plain film revealing widened joint space and osteopenia consistent with septic arthritis of hip.

Several radiographic studies can be used in the further evaluation of pediatric osteomyelitis. Radionucleotide bone scan has been a traditional exam that shows increased uptake around infected bone (Fig. 2.3). There is increasing experience using magnetic resonance imaging (MRI) in visualizing infected bone and bone marrow for the diagnosis of osteomyelitis. In centers in which there is expertise in the use of MRI, it is often a front-line study. It should be noted that MRI is sensitive, but not specific. Although it is very helpful in documenting abnormalities in bone, bone marrow, or soft tissue, it is not specific in determining the etiology of these changes. Appearance of bone and bone marrow in infection, trauma, or even infarction following sickle cell crisis can appear similar. Interpretation of MRI findings should always be done with the clinical context in mind (Figs. 2.4 and 2.5).

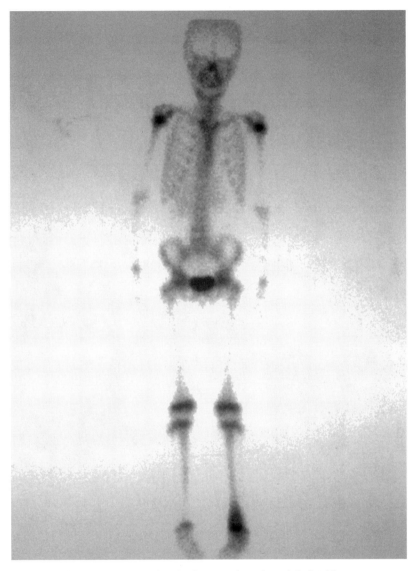

FIG. 2.3. Bone scan showing increased uptake at left distal femur.

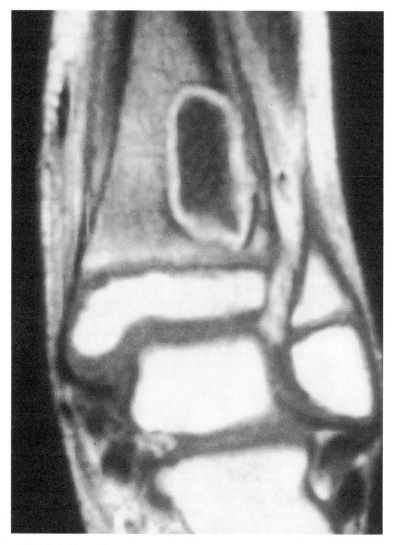

FIG. 2.4. Magnetic resonance image revealing large abscess in distal tibia.

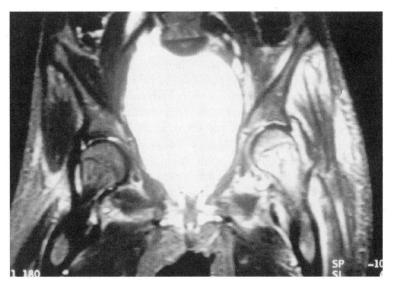

FIG. 2.5. Magnetic resonance image revealing osteomyelitis of left femoral head.

MANAGEMENT

All Patients with Bacterial Arthritis of the Hip Require Prompt Surgical Drainage and Irrigation

The presence of fluid as seen by ultrasound in the correct clinical setting necessitates immediate aspiration of that fluid. This can be done by either orthopedic surgery or interventional radiology under fluoroscopy. A joint aspirate that reveals greater than 100,000 white blood cells/m^3 is strongly correlated with septic arthritis. If the fluid is thought to be consistent with septic arthritis, the child should proceed immediately to the operating room for drainage. Because Gram stain and cultures are positive in only a small fraction of hip aspirates (25% to 30%), the decision to proceed to surgical drainage is determined by the cell count profile of the aspirated fluid.

Antibiotic Therapy for Pediatric Osteomyelitis

After the diagnosis of pediatric osteomyelitis is made, empiric therapy is begun. The major organism for pediatric osteomyelitis is *S. aureus*. It is increasingly appreciated that a large proportion of community-acquired *S. aureus* is methicillin resistant. Once seen only as a nosocomial infection, some communities report that up to 70% of *S. au-*

reus infections are resistant to methicillin. When confronted with *S. aureus* disease, the pediatrician can no longer assume that the organism will be sensitive to traditional antistaphylococcal medications such as nafcillin or first-generation cephalosporins. Community-acquired methicillin-resistant *S. aureus* (MRSA) is often sensitive to clindamycin and trimethoprim-sulfamethoxazole. Some clinicians are now empirically using clindamycin for initial treatment of community-acquired *S. aureus* disease; this usually covers both methicillin-susceptible and methicillin-resistant strains.

Although community-acquired MRSA is often initially susceptible to clindamycin, it has been noted that MRSA sensitive to clindamycin but resistant to erythromycin has the potential to develop clindamycin resistance. The specific test for the presence of inducible clindamycin resistance is the erythromycin induction (D) test. Although it is known that D-testing can detect inducible clindamycin resistance in a large percentage of MRSA isolates, it is not clear whether this *in vitro* test predicts clinical failure of clindamycin. There are scattered case reports of actual clinical failure in patients with a positive D test in whom clindamycin was used; it is advised that long-term clindamycin treatment for MRSA, such as that given for osteomyelitis, be approached with caution. Alternatives for long-term antibiotic therapy for MRSA infections include vancomycin and linezolid.

Before the development of the *Haemophilus influenzae* vaccine, this organism was also a frequent cause of pediatric osteomyelitis and septic arthritis. Despite the decline in *H. influenzae* disease, gram-negative organisms still play a role in pediatric osteomyelitis. *K. kingae*, a fastidious hemolytic gram-negative bacilli, has emerged in recent years as an invasive pathogen in children. Osteomyelitis and septic arthritis are the most common presentations of invasive *K. kingae* infections in children. Recent studies have suggested that about 20% of septic arthritis and osteomyelitis may be due to this organism. Some series have reported that *K. kingae* is the most common cause of septic arthritis in children younger than 2 years, being the causative agent in almost one half of cases. Thought to be a normal part of the oral flora in children, this pathogen gains access to the bloodstream in a manner similar to *S. aureus*. It is postulated that disruption of the respiratory or oral mucosa allows colonizing bacteria to enter the bloodstream. Preceding stomatitis is thought to play a role in the development of bacteremia and subsequent infection. Bone infection caused by *K. kingae* can be present in unusual locations, such as metatarsal bones and the epiphysis of long bones. *Kingella* is a fastidious aerobic pathogen that may not grow on standard agar; direct inoculation of an osteoarticular aspirate into blood culture bottles has been reported to improve the yield of cultures. Polymerase chain reaction amplification of synovial fluid has also been employed successfully in identifying the organism. *K. kingae* remains highly susceptible to many antibiotics, including third-generation cephalosporins.

Salmonella species are other gram-negative organisms that can cause osteomyelitis, particularly in patients with sickle cell anemia. It is for this reason that therapy with clindamycin, nafcillin, or a first-generation cephalosporin, combined with a third-generation cephalosporin (for optimal gram-negative coverage), is often used as empiric treatment of osteomyelitis until culture results are available.

Duration of Therapy

Early studies pointed to a higher relapse rate in patients treated for 3 weeks or less. Chronic infection has also been reported to develop more frequently in patients receiving only 3 weeks of therapy as compared with patients receiving therapy for 4 weeks or longer. Many clinicians believe that the minimum duration of treatment is 4 weeks and often continue treatment for as long as 6 weeks.

The monitoring of therapy using the sedimentation rate and C-reactive protein has been advocated. In children with septic arthritis, it is thought that the serum C-reactive protein peaks within 48 hours after treatment and normalizes in about 1 week. In contrast, the sedimentation rate may continue to increase despite effective treatment until day 5 and may remain elevated for more than 1 month. It has been recommended that the C-reactive protein be measured about 2 days after treatment is begun. Normalization suggests effective therapy.

Treatment is often continued until the sedimentation rate returns to normal values; this usually coincides with about a 1-month duration of therapy. An increasing C-reactive protein level or persistently elevated sedimentation rate can herald the need for surgical drainage. If, after 1 month of therapy, the repeated sedimentation rate is greater than 30 mm/h, a repeat MRI can be obtained to determine the need for surgery. Antibiotics can then continue for an additional 3 weeks, with repeat MRI and sedimentation rate done at that time.

Intravenous versus Oral Antibiotics

Traditionally, it was thought that serious bacterial infections such as osteomyelitis required intravenous antibiotics. In the early 1980s, studies examined the efficacy of oral treatment of pediatric osteomyelitis. These studies used the serum bactericidal titer (SBT) or Schlichter's test. This test is a modification of the MIC test. Patients with proven *S. aureus* osteomyelitis are given high-dose oral therapy, often 100 mg/kg per day of oral cephalexin. Serial dilutions are made from peak and trough serum samples. To these serial dilutions, an aliquot of the patient's infecting organism is added; the dilutions remaining clear after 24 hours of incubation is then plated on agar plates. The dilution at which bacteria fail to grow on agar plates is the peak and trough bactericidal titer (Fig. 2.6).

Prospective studies have determined that children with acute hematogenous osteomyelitis with a peak SBT of greater than or equal to 1:16 and a trough of greater than or equal to 1:2 achieve bacteriologic and clinical cure. Following these studies, many physicians advocate the use of oral antibiotics if the following conditions are met: (a) an organism is isolated, (b) adequate peak and trough SBTs can be obtained on oral therapy, and (c) compliance with oral therapy can be assured.

During the past 5 years, numerous reports have questioned the necessity of SBTs during oral therapy for osteomyelitis. Small series have reported good outcome in patients treated with oral antibiotics without confirmatory SBT measurement. To this day, there is great variation in clinical practice; some institutions will not use oral therapy unless a pathogen is isolated and adequate SBTs can be documented.

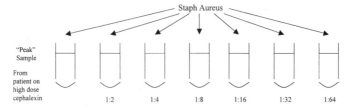

Serial dilutions made and bacterial aliquots added to each tube.

After 24 hours, 1:16 tube is cloudy, concentration dilution fails to inhibit bacterial growth.

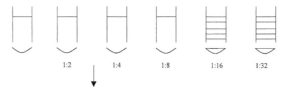

Tubes which show inhibition then plated on agar. Bacteria grow on 1:8 dilution but not on 1:4

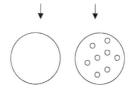

FIG. 2.6. Serum bactericidal titer (Schlichter's test) evaluating oral antibiotic treatment of *Staphylococcus aureus* osteomyelitis.

Some clinicians use oral therapy only if they are sure of the infecting organism, but do not think that SBTs are necessary. It is likely that the pediatrician caring for a child with osteomyelitis will have to make a case-by-case decision regarding what is the best mode of treatment for that particular child.

Antibiotic Therapy for Pediatric Septic Arthritis

Septic arthritis in joints other than the hip may not require surgical intervention, although repeated aspirations are sometimes used if fluid reaccumulates. Failure of septic arthritis to respond to appropriate antibiotic therapy should always lead to the consideration for surgical drainage. As in osteomyelitis, antibiotic therapy is traditionally given for at least 4 weeks. As in osteomyelitis, there is increasing experience in switching patients to oral antibiotic therapy after their physical exam has normalized. Many centers use an SBT with a peak titer of 1:16 as the level correlated with bacteriologic eradication and clinical cure.

Chronic Osteomyelitis

Although the increased duration of effective therapy has reduced the risk for chronic osteomyelitis, chronic infection can occur and can be difficult to treat. Organisms can survive in bone, and the accompanying bone necrosis may limit antibiotic penetration into infected areas. Although acute hematogenous osteomyelitis is typically treated with medical therapy alone, chronic disease often requires both medical and surgical treatment. Aggressive surgical techniques, which involve complete débridement of necrotic bone as well as the creation of muscle flaps for revascularization, are often required.

There remains no consensus on the duration of antibiotic therapy for chronic osteomyelitis. If at all possible, medical therapy should be dictated by the results of culture obtained at the time of surgery. Treatment courses of 3 to 6 months are reported to be generally effective.

Management of Pediatric Osteomyelitis and Septic Arthritis

1. Pathogens
   a. *Staphylococcus* aureus (including methicillin-resistant strains)
   b. *Salmonella* species (found in patients with sickle cell anemia)
   c. *Kingella kingae*
2. Initial treatment
   a. Clindamycin, 40 mg/kg per day in three divided doses, combined with Cefotaxime, 100 mg/kg per day; or ceftriaxone, 50 to 75 mg/kg per day
   b. For methicillin-sensitive *S. aureus,* consider switching to high-dose cephalexin (100 mg/kg per day) once the patient is afebrile and clinically improved. Demonstration of peak SBT of more than 1:16 correlates with clinical and microbiologic cure.

SELECTED READINGS

Kallio MJ, Unkila-Kallio L, Aalto K, et al. Serum C-reactive protein, erythrocyte sedimentation rate and white blood cell count in septic arthritis of children. *Pediatr Infect Dis J* 1997;(16)4:411–413.

Karwowska A, Davies HD, Jadarji T. Epidemiology and outcome of osteomyelitis in the era of sequential intravenous: oral therapy. *Pediatr Infect Dis J* 1998;(17)11:1021–1026.

Kocher MS, Zurakowski D, Kasser JR. Differentiating between septic arthritis and transient synovitis of the hip in children: an evidence-based clinical prediction algorithm. *J Bone Joint Surg Am* 1999;81(12):1662–1670.

Martinez-Aguilar G, Hammerman W, Mason E, et al. Clindamycin treatment of invasive infections caused by community acquired, methicillin-resistant and methicillin-susceptible *Staphylococcus aureus* in children. *Pediatr Infect Dis J* 2003;22(7):593–599.

Moumile K, Merckx J, Glorion C, et al. Osteoarticular infections caused by *Kingella kingae* in children: contribution of polymerase chain reaction to the microbiologic diagnosis. *Pediatr Infect Dis J* 2003;22(9):837–839.

Newton PO, Ballock RT, Bradley JS. Oral antibiotic therapy of bacterial arthritis. *Pediatr Infect Dis J* 1999;(18)12:1102–1103.

Prober CG, Yeager AS. Use of the serum bactericidal titer to assess the adequacy of oral antibiotic therapy in the treatment of acute hematogenous osteomyelitis. *J Pediatr* 1979;95(1):131–135.

Yagupsky P, Dagan R. Kingella kingae: an emerging cause of invasive infections in children. *Clin Infect Dis* 1997;24(5):860–866.

3

Congenital Infections

BASIC CONSIDERATIONS

Infections can be transmitted from mother to developing fetus transplacentally, at the time of delivery, and through breast milk.

The diagnosis of congenital and perinatal infections is complicated by several issues:

1. Infected babies may be asymptomatic or minimally symptomatic when born, only to develop symptoms and disabilities in the following weeks, months, or even years.
2. Babies born symptomatic may have findings such as anemia, thrombocytopenia, jaundice, and microcephaly, which can be the result of infections with several different pathogens (e.g., cytomegalovirus [CMV], syphilis, rubella).
3. Laboratory evaluation for congenital and some perinatal infections has often included the use of TORCH titers (i.e., toxoplasmosis, rubella, CMV, and herpes). TORCH titers are immunoglobulin G (IgG) antibodies that readily cross the placenta and may persist for months in the neonatal circulation. As 50% of adults have serologic evidence of previous infection with CMV, herpes simplex virus, or toxoplasmosis, up to 50% of newborns tested will have positive TORCH titers for these organisms. TORCH titers are of no value in the diagnosis of congenital and perinatal infections. Rather, a disease-specific approach using precise clinical and laboratory methods is required.

CYTOMEGALOVIRUS

Epidemiology

CMV is the most common congenital infection, affecting 1% to 2% of all newborns. The rate of infection in a fetus of a mother with primary infection is between

40% and 50%; the rate of infection is less than 1% if the mother has reactivated infection. Most infected infants (90%) are asymptomatic at birth; only 10% of these children have long-term sequelae. The most common sequela is asymptomatic congenital CMV infection sensorineural hearing loss. This hearing loss can be progressive and may be unilateral or bilateral.

Presentation

Ten percent of infants with congenital CMV infection are symptomatic at birth. These patients often present with multiple organ system involvement, including intrauterine growth retardation, petechiae, anemia, leukopenia, and thrombocytopenia. A classic finding on computed tomography of the head in congenital CMV is periventricular calcification (Fig. 3.1). The predilection for the calcification in this area is believed to be related to the tendency of CMV to infect the rapidly dividing

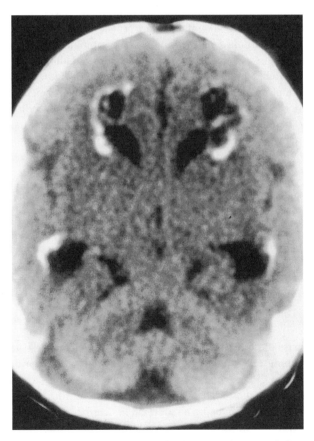

FIG. 3.1. Periventricular calcifications seen in congenital cytomegalovirus infection.

germinal matrix cells. Magnetic resonance imaging of neonates with congenital CMV infection may also reveal irregular areas in the junction of the gray and white matter, accompanied by the presence of ventricular pseudocysts. Patients with congenital CMV may have continual neurologic damage even after birth, which is thought to be secondary to persistent viral replication.

Diagnosis

The gold standard of diagnosis is isolation of the virus, usually from the urine. Urine viral cultures are often positive within days because the kidney is a principal site of viral replication. Proof of congenital infection is based on obtaining appropriate specimens within 3 weeks of birth. After this time, distinguishing between intrauterine infection and perinatal infection may be difficult.

Management

Patients with congenital CMV infection are at risk for a variety of disabilities, including developmental delay and hearing loss. Symptomatic children are considered to have the highest risk for long-term abnormalities, although recent longitudinal studies have found predicting disability difficult. It is known that the major disability in asymptomatic congenital CMV infection is sensorineural hearing loss. This hearing loss may be progressive in affected infants. After a diagnosis of congenital CMV is made, routine assessments should be instituted. It has been recommended that a careful ophthalmology exam be performed at 12 months, 3 years, and at entrance to preschool. Audiology examinations should be done every 3 months until 3 years of age and then annually.

Diagnosis of Cytomegalovirus

- Urine viral culture
- Hearing evaluation
- Ultrasound or computed tomograph of brain
- Eye examination

No definitive protocols exist for the treatment of congenital CMV infection. Clinical trials are in progress; a recent randomized clinical trial comparing outcomes in symptomatic infants given the antiviral agent ganciclovir with those in patients receiving no treatment suggested that there may be a benefit from treatment, the greatest benefit in treated children being a reduction in hearing loss. In early protocols of treatment of CMV, symptomatic infants were administered intravenous ganciclovir for 6 weeks; later studies extended treatment of affected infants with intravenous and then oral ganciclovir for up to 1 year. Currently, it is not recommended that asymptomatic infants found to be congenitally infected receive ganciclovir. These children should be followed carefully for the development of sensorineural hearing loss. Neonates with life-threatening symptomatic disease, including intractable thrombocytopenia, pneumonia, or hepatic failure, are candidates for antiviral therapy. It is my experience and the experience of investigators nationally that therapy can be very beneficial in these cases.

Complications of ganciclovir include difficulties in maintaining intravenous access and neutropenia. There will likely be continued efforts to identify precisely and treat those infants likely to have long-term sequelae from congenital CMV infection and those most likely to benefit from therapy.

HERPES SIMPLEX VIRUS

Epidemiology

Depending on the population surveyed, as many as 10% to 15% of women report a history of genital herpes. This number may actually be higher because many infected women do not have a history of visible genital lesions. Previously, pregnant women who reported a history of genital herpes had weekly viral cultures obtained as they approached delivery. However, when results of the viral cultures become available, typically in 7 days, they were of little value. This practice of weekly viral cultures has been replaced by a more basic approach; women who do not have active lesions at the time of delivery are often allowed to deliver vaginally.

The current practice is such that exposure to herpesvirus can never be avoided, and pediatricians must be vigilant to the various manifestations of neonatal herpes. The manifestations of neonatal herpes usually present in the first month of life.

Presentation

Mucocutaneous Disease

Herpetic vesicles can appear on the scalp, mouth, eyes, and skin. Although children with mucocutaneous disease may initially be well appearing, 75% progress to disseminated disease (Fig. 3.2).

Encephalitis

Encephalitis may present with lethargy, seizures, and a cerebrospinal pleocytosis that shows a lymphocytic predominance. In infants with meningitis or encephalitis, positive temporal lobe spikes on electroencephalogram (EEG) are found in 80% of cases and represent a noninvasive means of diagnosis. This is often misdiagnosed as aseptic meningitis or as the more common enteroviral meningitis. Aseptic meningitis in the first month of life should be considered herpes until proved otherwise.

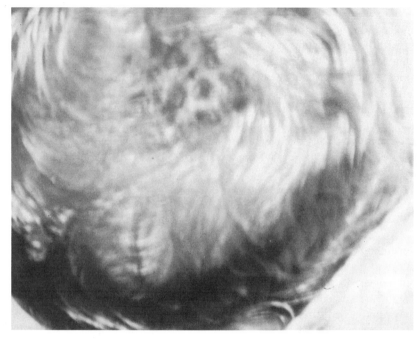

FIG. 3.2. Scalp vesicles in a 2-week-old infant representing mucocutaneous herpes infection (see color plate).

Pneumonia

Rarely, herpes can present with progressive pneumonia in the neonatal period. This is usually not associated with skin vesicles but can be associated with dissemination, with increased liver function tests, coagulopathy, and organ failure.

Disseminated Disease

Disseminated disease is often associated with fever, coagulopathy, and abnormalities of liver function tests. Vesicles are usually not present initially. Disseminated disease has a very high mortality rate, even when treated appropriately. A persistently febrile neonate, particularly if blood cultures remain negative and liver enzymes are elevated, should raise strong suspicion of herpes (Table 3.1).

Diagnosis

The first issue in diagnosis is a clinical suspicion of herpes simplex disease. Herpetic vesicles in the neonatal period are an emergency. If there is any suspicion regarding whether a skin lesion is a vesicle, empiric acyclovir should be started while appropriate studies are obtained. This is very similar to the management of the febrile

TABLE 3.1. *Neonatal Herpes: Clinical Manifestations*

Mucocutaneous disease (skin, eye, mouth)
  Groups of vesicles; a large percentage of untreated cases progress to disseminated disease
  Diagnosis: Direct immunofluorescence or viral culture of vesicles
Encephalitis
  Presents with lethargy, seizures at 2 to 3 weeks of age
  Cerebrospinal fluid reveals 100 to 200 white cells with lymphocytic predominance
  Diagnosis: Viral culture (positive in <20%)
  Polymerase chain reaction of cerebrospinal fluid
  Electroencephalogram reveals temporal lobe spikes in 80%
Pneumonia
  Vesicles typically not present
  Progressive pulmonary infiltrates
  Negative bacterial cultures
  Elevation of liver function tests
Disseminated disease
  Fever, lethargy
  Negative bacterial cultures
  Elevated liver function tests, coagulopathy
  Vesicles typically absent
Diagnosis: viral cultures, polymerase chain reaction of blood, cerebrospinal fluid

neonate, in whom empiric antibiotics are started until blood cultures are final. Aseptic meningitis in the neonate should also be considered herpes until proved otherwise.

There are several ways of making the diagnosis of neonatal herpes. Vesicles can be scraped to obtain viral culture and tested for direct fluorescent antibodies; these have relatively high yield. Polymerase chain reaction (PCR) of the serum and spinal fluid is now considered the gold standard for diagnosis. Even in neonates with only mucocutaneous disease, the rate of a positive serum PCR can be greater than 50%. There are increasing reports of reduced sensitivity of cerebrospinal fluid (CSF) PCR in diagnosing pediatric herpes simplex encephalitis, particularly if CSF has been obtained on the first day of illness. In patients with a compatible clinical picture of herpes simplex encephalitis, particularly if an alternative diagnosis such as enterovirus has not been confirmed, it may be prudent to continue treatment until a second sample of CSF has been obtained and tested.

Management

Treatment of neonatal herpes is intravenous acyclovir. Herpes simplex disease in the neonate is never treated either empirically or definitively with topical or oral acyclovir. The dose is 60 mg/kg per day in three divided doses. The treatment duration is 14 days for mucocutaneous disease and 21 days for disseminated disease or in neonates in whom central nervous system (CNS) involvement is suspected. Supportive care in terms of controlling seizures and coagulopathy is also critical in the management of these patients.

Herpes simplex virus is a latent virus, and it is assumed that most neonates with infection will develop latent infection. There is ongoing concern that reactivation of latent virus in infants with a history of neonatal infection may be associated with continued morbidity. Children with a history of mucocutaneous disease often have recurrences of their vesicles; the effect of this on long-term development is uncertain. Studies conducted at the National Institute of Allergy and Infectious Disease have found that infants with more than three recurrences of mucocutaneous vesicles have a higher incidence of neurologic sequelae. It is postulated that cutaneous reactivation may be associated with subclinical reactivation in the CNS.

There have been initial clinical trials to enroll children with recurrent cutaneous herpes on long-term oral acyclovir therapy given at 300 mg/m^2 per dose two or three times daily for 6 months. Although this does seem to prevent herpes recurrences, nearly half of the children develop neutropenia, defined as white blood cell counts of less than 1,000/m^3. Currently, there is no consensus regarding preventative therapy; this should be answered in the future by prospective clinical trials.

Diagnosis of Herpes Simplex Virus

- Direct immunofluorescent antibodies (DFA), viral culture of vesicles
- Serum, CSF PCR
- EEG (80% show temporal lobe spikes)

CONGENITAL SYPHILIS

Epidemiology

Congenital syphilis results from inadequate or late treatment of syphilis in a pregnant woman. Infection passed to the newborn can result in stillbirth, symptomatic neonatal disease, or infection that does not manifest until later in childhood.

Presentation

Infected infants may appear normal at birth, only to manifest symptoms in the first year of life. These infants may present with mucocutaneous lesions, anemia, and organomegaly. Congenital syphilis nephrotic syndrome or an osteochondritis that causes decreased movement of the affected extremity (pseudoparalysis of Parrot) may be seen. Late manifestations of congential syphilis include interstitial keratitis and notching of the central incisors (Hutchinson's teeth).

Evaluation

There are two types of serologic tests used for the diagnosis of syphilis in adults. The nontreponemal tests include the VDRL and RPR. These can be quantitated by titers and, after successful therapy, usually become nonreactive. The treponemal tests, which include MHA-TP and FTA-ABS, are not quantitative and are thought to remain positive for life. All syphilis serology crosses the placenta and, like other TORCH titers, cannot be used for diagnosis in neonates. Because an infected infant may be asymptomatic at birth (only to develop the disease in later life), we therefore have an unusual situation in which both laboratory tests and physical examination are not helpful in the diagnosis of congenital syphilis.

In the early 1990s, new criteria were established for the presumptive diagnosis of congenital syphilis. An infant born to a mother considered untreated or inadequately treated receives the presumptive diagnosis of congenital syphilis. The definition of inadequate maternal treatment includes the following:

- Syphilis during pregnancy treated with a nonpenicillin regimen, such as erythromycin
- Syphilis during pregnancy treated with an appropriate penicillin regimen without the expected posttherapy decrease in nontreponemal titers
- Syphilis treated less than 1 month before delivery
- Syphilis treated before pregnancy but with insufficient serologic follow-up to assess the response to treatment

Some investigators believe that the rate of fetal infection from a mother with secondary syphilis in pregnancy is so high that treatment should also be considered for all those infants as well.

Children with a presumptive diagnosis of congenital syphilis should have the following evaluation:

- Physical exam, although it should be stressed that infected infants appear be normal at birth
- Nontreponemal and treponemal tests done from infant blood rather than cord blood
- CSF for cells, protein, and VDRL
- Complete blood count and platelet count
- Long-bone radiographs looking for osteolytic lesions

A major part of the evaluation for congenital syphilis in the infant includes the evaluation for congenital neurosyphilis. The diagnosis of congenital neurosyphilis is important because several forms of penicillin, including penicillin G benzathine, do not reach treponicidal concentrations in the CSF. The gold standard for CNS disease is the rabbit infectivity test. This test involves the inoculation of clinical specimens into rabbits and is sensitive enough to detect as few as 10 organisms. Unfortunately, this test is not routinely available outside research laboratories.

Controversy continues about the best diagnostic approach to document CNS involvement in congenital syphilis. Recently, PCR of blood and CSF, in addition to IgM immunoblotting, has been developed. Compared with the rabbit infectivity test, these studies were found to identify 94% and 100% of infants with CNS disease, respectively. It is hoped that these tests will become widely available in the future. In infants with otherwise normal clinical, laboratory, and radiographic studies, CNS involvement is unusual.

Diagnosis of Neonatal Syphilis

- Maternal history
- Long bone films
- Serum, CSF VDRL
- Complete blood count

Management

Asymptomatic infants who have normal CSF results, complete blood counts, and radiographic examination (and therefore low likelihood of CNS involvement) may be treated with a single dose of intramuscular benzathine penicillin at a dose of 50,000 units/kg. Neonates who have abnormalities on physical exam or laboratory evaluation should be treated with aqueous penicillin G, 100,000 to 150,000 units/kg per day administered at 50,000 units/kg per dose intravenously every 12 hours for the first 7 days of life and every 8 hours thereafter for a total of 10 days. An additional option for these patients with proven or highly probable disease includes procaine penicillin, 50,000 units/kg per dose given intramuscularly once a day for 10 days.

Follow-up is critical in infants treated for congenital syphilis. Serologic nontreponemal tests should be performed 3, 6, and 12 months after conclusion of treatment. Nontreponemal titers should be nonreactive by 6 months of age if treatment was adequate. Children with increasing titers or persistent stable titers should be considered for repeat treatment.

CONGENITAL RUBELLA

Epidemiology

Congenital rubella infection is unusual because the readily available vaccine prevents infection in mothers of childbearing age. However, cases still occur in populations that are not optimally vaccinated. Most cases of congenital rubella are the result of primary maternal disease during pregnancy. The risk for fetal infection is highest during early gestation, although the most severe manifestations occur when infection is in the last trimester.

Presentation

Patients born with congenital rubella usually suffer from severe intrauterine growth retardation as well as a variety of cardiac, ophthalmologic, and neurologic defects. The most common congenital heart defects include patent ductus arteriosus and pulmonary artery stenosis. Cataracts occur in more than 30% of cases. Severe cases often have "celery stalk" appearance of long bones visible on plain radiographs. Organomegaly, thrombocytopenia, and purpuric skin lesions may also be seen. There is considerable clinical overlap in patients with congenital CMV. As with many congenital infections, many children may be asymptomatic at birth but develop manifestations later in life.

Diagnosis

Diagnosis is made by detection of rubella-specific serum IgM antibodies. Congenital infection can also be diagnosed by documenting increasing serum concentrations of infant rubella IgG over several months. Virus is readily excreted from throat, urine, and CSF, but viral isolation of rubella is difficult and usually not achieved.

Diagnosis of Congenital Rubella

- Rubella IgM
- Persistence of IgG
- Viral culture of throat, urine, CSF

Management

At the present time, there is no treatment for infants with congenital rubella. Defects of the eyes are managed as needed. Contact isolation is recommended for children with proven or presumed congenital rubella during the first year of life.

CONGENITAL TOXOPLASMOSIS

Epidemiology

Congenital toxoplasmosis occurs when a woman acquires primary infection during pregnancy. Overall transmission rate is between 20% and 30%. The rate of transmission is low when women are infected in the first trimester, but when infection occurs during this time, infants are more severely affected. Conversely, if infections occur later in pregnancy, the risk for transmission is high, but infected infants are less likely to have the most severe clinical features of the disease.

Studies have found that most causes of toxoplasmosis in humans include eating rare to medium cooked beef, working in an outside environment, and cat exposure. In some cases, the actual source of transmission remains unclear despite repeated investigation. Factors that predict congenital toxoplasmosis have been found to include mother's birth outside the United States, multiparity, and the level of education of the mother (the least and most educated appear to be at highest risk).

Presentation

The classical clinical triad of congenital toxoplasmosis includes retinitis, hydrocephalus, and intracranial calcification, although this is present in only a small

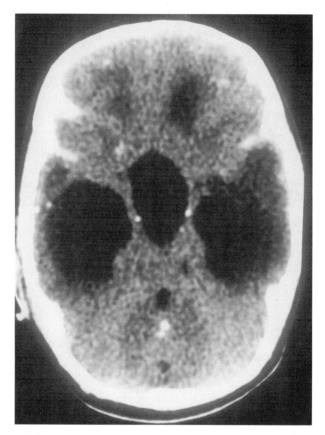

FIG. 3.3. Hydrocephalous, intracranial calcifications seen in congenital toxoplasmosis.

number of cases (Fig. 3.3). Congenital toxoplasmosis is usually asymptomatic at birth. As they grow older, a significant percentage of these children have learning disabilities, visual impairment, or mental retardation.

Evaluation

Traditional TORCH titers are again of little value in the diagnosis of congenital toxoplasmosis. Maternal IgG antibodies cross the placenta and are positive in a good percentage of newborns. Commercially available IgM assays are not recommended for routine use because they have very high false-positive and false-negative rates. The reference laboratory at the Palo Alto Medical Foundation, under the direction of Dr. Jack Remington, is the standard way of making the laboratory diagnosis of congenital toxoplasmosis (Palo Alto Medical Foundation; telephone number 650–853–4828.) This laboratory performs a variety of specialized assays, including the following:

Sabin Feldman dye test. This test measures primarily IgG antibodies. Any titer is considered positive.

Immunosorbent agglutination assay (IgM-ISAgA). This test is highly sensitive and recommended for infants in whom congenital toxoplasmosis is suspected.

IgA enzyme-linked immunosorbent assay (ELISA). This test is actually more sensitive for detection of infection in newborns than the IgM assay. Both tests are done if congenital toxoplasmosis is suspected.

Evaluation of infants with suspected congenital toxoplasmosis should also include ophthalmologic examination and computed tomography or ultrasound of the brain to determine whether hydrocephalus or calcifications are present.

Diagnosis of Neonatal Toxoplasmosis

- Ophthalmology exam
- Ultrasound, computed tomography of brain
- Toxoplasmosis IgA, IgM by "double-sandwich" ELISA

Management of Confirmed Congenital Toxoplasmosis

Infants who are diagnosed with congenital toxoplasmosis require treatment. The therapy for congenital toxoplasmosis is as follows:

Sulfadiazine, 100 mg/mL; half of child's weight (in kilograms) equals number of mls, given twice a day

Pyrimethamine, 2 mg/mL; half of child's weight (in kilograms) equals number of mls, given once a day

Folinic acid (leucovorin) 5-mg tablets, 2 tablets crushed in formula Monday, Wednesday, and Friday

For all infants with both asymptomatic and symptomatic congenital infection, therapy is recommended for 1 year.

Diagnosis of Acute Toxoplasmosis in Pregnant Women

Diagnosis of toxoplasmosis in pregnancy is difficult because most patients have minimal symptoms; a mononucleosis-like illness or posterior cervical adenitis is sometimes seen. In women at increased risk for primary toxoplasmosis, screening for IgG antibodies can be performed. It is important to confirm all screenings with follow-up testing at a reference laboratory. The panel of testing available can often give an estimate of the timing of maternal infection.

If the mother has had primary infection during pregnancy, fetal infection can be evaluated using PCR of amniotic fluid. Serial ultrasound examinations looking for hydrocephalus, organomegaly, and intracranial calcifications are used to determine whether fetal infection is causing specific organ system disease. Maternal antitoxoplasmosis treatment is frequently given in this situation because it may reduce fetal damage.

LYMPHOCYTIC CHORIOMENINGITIS VIRUS

Epidemiology

Lymphocytic choriomeningitis virus (LCMV) is a single-stranded RNA virus that causes chronic infection in house mice and pet hamsters, which then shed the virus in the urine and feces. Humans may be infected by direct contact with excreta or aerosolization of viral particles.

Presentation

It has become increasingly appreciated that LCMV may cause a congenital infection characterized by periventricular calcification, hydrocephalus, and chorioretinitis. This may give a symptom complex similar to other congenital infections, particularly toxoplasmosis or CMV.

Diagnosis

The true incidence of LCMV congenital infection is not known because it is likely that only the most extreme cases are diagnosed. The diagnosis should be considered in the neonate with intracranial calcifications or hydrocephalous, especially if the workup for toxoplasmosis and CMV are negative. Diagnosis is by immuno-fluorescent antibody or ELISA.

Management

At the present time, there is no therapy for LCMV. Because of this newly described syndrome, expectant mothers should be cautioned regarding contact with mice and other rodents.

HUMAN IMMUNODEFICIENCY VIRUS

Epidemiology

A pregnant woman with untreated human immunodeficiency virus (HIV) has an approximately 20% to 25% chance of giving birth to an infected infant. HIV can be transmitted transplacentally at any stage of the pregnancy. Most infants are infected at the time of delivery by exposure to maternal blood and body fluids. HIV can also be transmitted during the postnatal period through breast-feeding.

HIV antibody crosses the placenta; thus, 100% of infants born to HIV-positive women are HIV antibody positive. Maternal HIV antibody can persist in the child for up to 18 months. The only certain statement regarding an HIV antibody–positive infant is that the mother is infected.

Presentation

There are numerous presentations of the child with HIV infection. Some children present in the first year of life with severe thrush, organomegaly, and failure to thrive. *Pneumocystis jiroveci* (formerly *P. carinii*), in a previously thriving infant is a classic presentation and should always be considered in a child who suddenly develops severe interstitial pneumonia and respiratory failure. A subset of children with HIV infection remain relatively well for years, with the only signs being isolated developmental delay or thrombocytopenia.

Diagnosis

Diagnosis of HIV infection in the infant is made by serum HIV PCR. This test is obtained at 1 and 4 months of age. If these tests are negative, the child is assumed uninfected. Positive test at this time indicates that true infection is likely. Some clinicians follow infants for up to 18 months to document seroreversion to HIV-negative antibody status.

Ongoing efforts continue to reduce mother-to-child transmission. In 1994, AIDS Clinical Trial Group (ACTG) 076 was developed. In this protocol, zidovudine (AZT) was given to the mother starting in the second trimester of pregnancy. During delivery, intravenous AZT was given to the mother. After delivery, AZT suspension (10 mg/mL) was given at a dose of 2 mg/kg every 6 hours for 6 weeks. The transmission rate in this study dropped from 25% to 8%; the study was stopped early because the statistically and clinically significant findings could not ethically be kept from the control arm of the study.

During the past 10 years, the development of highly active antiretroviral therapy (HAART) has led to further reduction in mother-to-child transmission. Strong consideration for elective cesarean section is given, particularly if maternal viral load exceeds 5,000 copies/mL. Intravenous AZT continues to be given at time of delivery. After delivery, oral AZT is given to the child for 6 weeks. The 10 mg/mL suspension is given at a dose of 2 mg/kg orally every 6 hours. Currently, the incidence of transmission under these aggressive protocols is less than 2%. It is likely that further refinements to reduce maternal transmission (including additional drugs administered to the infant) will be developed. Maternal transmission of HIV to infants should be considered a highly preventable condition. All pregnant women should be counseled about HIV testing. This ensures the diagnosis of women unaware of their infection and protection of their unborn children.

Management

If effective protocols for prevention of maternal transmissions are used, transmission of HIV from mother to child should be less than 2%. The diagnosis of true HIV infection is made by PCR, showing viral copies of HIV at 1 and 4 months of age. If this indeed is documented, HIV infection is considered to have occurred in the infant. Protocols for the management of infant HIV infection are continually revised. Most specialist agree that HAART therapy should be given once infant HIV infection has been documented. Although monotherapy is used in the protocols preventing maternal transmission, for actual treatment of confirmed disease, combination of at least three antiretroviral drugs should be considered.

SELECTED READINGS

Azimi PH, Janner D, Berne P, et al. Concentrations of procaine and aqueous penicillin in the cerebrospinal fluid of infants treated for congenital syphilis. *J Pediatr* 1994;124(4):649–653.

Bale JF. Congenital infections. *Neurol Clin* 2002:20(4):1039–1060.

Bechtel RT, Haught KA, Mets MB. Lymphocytic choriomeningitis virus: a new addition to the TORCH evaluation. *Arch Ophthalmol* 1997;115(5):680–681.

Boyer KM. Diagnostic testing for congenital toxoplasmosis. *Pediatr Infect Dis J* 2001;20(1):59–60.

Litwin CM, Hill HR. Serologic and DNA-based testing for congenital and perinatal infections. *Pediatr Infect Dis J* 1997;16(12):1166–1175.

McAuley J, Boyer KM, Patel D, et al. Early and longitudinal evaluations of treated infants and children and untreated historical patients with congenital toxoplasmosis: the Chicago Collaborative Treatment Trial. *Clin Infect Dis* 1994;18(1)38–72.

Michaels MG, Greenberg DP, Sabo DL, et al. Treatment of children with congenital cytomegalovirus infection with ganciclovir. *Pediatr Infect Dis J* 2003;22(6):504–509.

Michelow IC, Wendel GD, Norgard MV, et al. Central nervous system infection in congenital syphilis. *N Engl J Med* 2002;346(23):1792–1798.

4

Congenital Immunodeficiencies

BASIC CONSIDERATIONS

Pediatricians who manage serious pediatric infections must often address a basic question:

> Is this infection the result of bad luck (i.e., when bad bacteria meet good children), or is it the result of an underlying immune problem?

PRIMARY IMMUNODEFICIENCIES

Epidemiology

The identification of primary immunodeficiencies in children is critical. A child with an unrecognized immunodeficiency may expire from an overwhelming opportunistic infection. Even when not fatal, multiple pneumonias in such patients can progress to chronic, debilitating pulmonary disease. Children with underlying immunodeficiency are also susceptible to adverse reactions if administered live vaccinations. It is important that the pediatrician consider the possibility of underlying immunodeficiency when managing serious infections in the first year of life.

The average child can have between six and eight respiratory infections per year. This number can increase if there are additional risk factors, such as attendance at day care, sibling exposures, or atopic disease. Although parents may complain that their child is "always sick," these infections are usually self-limited upper respiratory infections.

Age-related Clinical Patterns for Primary Immunodeficiencies

The immunodeficiencies involving T cells, such as severe combined immunodeficiency (SCID) or DiGeorge's syndrome, appear at an earlier age. These defects often present in the first 6 months of life with failure to thrive, diarrhea, pneumonia, and thrush. Significant lymphopenia is often seen. Antibody deficiency disease, such as X-linked agammaglobulinemia (Bruton's disease) often clinically manifest as maternal immunoglobulin levels wane after 6 months of age. Immunoglobulin deficiencies typically present with severe recurrent bacterial respiratory infections.

Presentation

It can be a considerable challenge for the primary care physician to distinguish the immunologically normal child having recurrent viral infections from the child who may have a primary immunodeficiency that requires specific diagnosis and therapy.

There has been an attempt to devise criteria for the evaluation of primary immunodeficiencies, often referred to as "red flags."

Signs of Primary Immunodeficiency

- A family history of primary immunodeficiency
- Infections with unusual organisms, such as *P. jiroveci* (formally *carinii*), which are so rare in the normal host that their presence always warrants an immune evaluation
- Recurrent deep-seated bacterial infections such as sepsis, osteomyelitis, or meningitis
- Increased number or severity of routine infections. Although this can be difficult to quantitate, greater than eight episodes of otitis media or two serious infections in the course of a year have been suggested as cutoffs.
- Failure to thrive in the first year of life
- Persistent oral thrush or mucocutaneous fungal infections after the first year of life
- Poor growth and development between infections

Diagnosis

Once a decision to screen for primary immunodeficiency is made, the following can be helpful laboratory screen:
- Measurement of serum immunoglobulin levels, including immunoglobulin E (IgE)
- Quantification of specific antibody responses to vaccination
- Absolute lymphocyte count
- T-cell numbers: (CD3, CD4, CD8) and B-cell numbers (CD19, CD20)
- *In vitro* lymphocyte proliferation tests (T cell function)
- Total complement levels (CH50)
- Nitroblue tetrazolium test (NBT)

Screening labs which come back abnormal, particularly in the correct clinical context, warrant referral to a pediatric immunologist or infectious disease specialist.

SPECIFIC PRIMARY IMMUNODEFICIENCIES

X-linked Agammaglobulinemia

Epidemiology and Etiology

Bruton's agammaglobulinemia is a pure B-cell immunodeficiency with a prevalence of 1 in 100,000 male children. Fifty percent of cases lack a family history and are thought to be the result of a spontaneous mutation. The cause of Bruton's agammaglobulinemia is a series of heterogenous mutations in the Bruton's tyrosine kinase (*BTK*) gene, which is on the long arm of the X chromosome at locus q21.3. The result of these heterogenous mutations is an arrest of B-cell maturation by the defective production of a tyrosine kinase protein. Affected individuals are unable to generate immunoglobulins.

Presentation

X-linked agammaglobulinemia is characterized by recurrent sinopulmonary infections with pyogenic organisms, notably *Haemophilus influenzae, Staphylococcus aureus*, and *Streptococcus pneumoniae*. Infections typically occur after the age of 6 months when maternal antibody levels fall. *Pseudomonas* species or staphylococcal sepsis associated with neutropenia has also been described as a presenting symptom. Chronic *Giardia* species infection and chronic enteroviral meningitis and meningoencephalitis are also well documented in this condition. *Ureaplasma urealyticum* has been reported as a cause of septic arthritis and chronic osteomyelitis in patients with Bruton's agammaglobulinemia.

A major clinical clue in patients with Bruton's agammaglobulinemia is the paucity of cervical lymph nodes and tonsillar tissues; patients with a history of recurrent otitis media or sinusitis should have a careful evaluation of lymphoid tissue.

Diagnosis

Diagnosis of Bruton's agammaglobulinemia is made by measurement of quantitative immunoglobulins as well as quantitation of circulating CD19 cells (B cells). Typically, patients have IgG levels of less than 200 mg/dL and no circulating B cells. Bruton's patients also typically do not make appropriate antibodies after routine immunizations. Assays for mutations in the *BTK* genes are done at research facilities and are not widely available.

Management

Treatment is the replacement of antibodies with intravenous immunoglobulin using 400 mg/kg per dose every 4 weeks. The goal is to maintain an IgG level of greater than 500 mg/dL.

X-linked (Burton's) Agammaglobulinemia

- Recurrent sinopulmonary infections
- *Pseudomonas* species sepsis
- Chronic enteroviral encephalitis

Hyper-IgM Syndrome

Epidemiology and Etiology

This syndrome usually has X-linked inheritance, but autosomal forms are occasionally seen. Patients with hyper-IgM syndrome have low levels of IgG and elevated levels of IgM. The cause of the condition is a defective or deficient CD40 ligand, a type 2 transmembrane glycoprotein. This protein is involved in the activation of B cells as well as in T-cell activation on monocytes and macrophages.

Presentation

Children with this condition present with chronic pyogenic infections similar to hypogammaglobulinemia patients. They are also susceptible to a variety of infections usually characteristic of T-cell immunodeficiency.

For patients younger than 1 year of age, the most common clinical presentation is *Pneumocystis jiroveci* (PCP) infection.

Diagnosis

The high rate of *P. jiroveci* is a distinct feature of X-linked hyper-IgM syndrome and should be strongly considered in an HIV-negative child with PCP and hypogammaglobulinemia. Chronic diarrhea and failure to thrive are also frequently encountered in these patients.

Management

Survival for this condition is poor and has been reported to be as low as 20% at 25 years of age. The mainstay of therapy is monthly intravenous immune globulin (IVIG) and PCP prophylaxis. There is increasing enthusiasm for bone marrow transplantation as a curative therapy.

Hyper-IgM Syndrome

- Low immunoglobulin with elevated IgM levels
- *Pneumocystis pneumonia*
- Pyogenic infection
- Chronic *Giardia* species infection
- Defective or absent CD40 ligand

DiGeorge's Syndrome

Epidemiology and Etiology

DiGeorge's syndrome is a congenital condition that results from alterations occurring during development of the third and fourth pharyngeal pouches. DiGeorge's syndrome is characterized by unusual facial features, congenital heart disease, and hypocalcemia.

Presentation

Most children with DiGeorge's syndrome who have heart defects show a chromosomal 22Q11 deletion. It is becoming apparent that the 22Q11 deletion syndrome includes not only DiGeorge's syndrome but also velocardiofacial syndrome. This deletion syndrome also has a large variability in expression; defects can include cardiac abnormalities, characteristic facial features, hypoparathyroidism, and cleft palate abnormalities.

Diagnosis

The test for DiGeorge's syndrome is a Fluorescence in situ hybridization (FISH) test on chromosome 22. This test should be considered in a patient with congenital heart disease (particularly abnormalities of the aortic arch) that is accompanied by unusual facial features and hypocalcemia.

DiGeorge's anomaly can also be associated with significant immunodeficiency. The initial description focused on severe T-cell immunodeficiency, although this is now considered rare, with an incidence of less than 2%. Despite the rarity of pure T-cell immunodeficiency, there is a considerable spectrum of immunodeficiency in patients with DiGeorge's syndrome.

A major issue in the evaluation of DiGeorge's syndrome is to identify those patients who will have persistence of profoundly depressed T-cell immune function.

It is believed that patients with "complete" DiGeorge's syndrome (severe T-cell immunodeficiency) do not improve spontaneously and are clinically similar to patients with severe combined immune deficiency. It has been recommended that the test of choice for determining the degree of T-cell immunodeficiency in DiGeorge's syndrome is the mitogen response; only patients with no mitogen response are considered to have the complete form.

Although T-cell immunodeficiency in DiGeorge's syndrome remains rare, it is increasingly appreciated that humoral immunodeficiency is relatively common. In some series, more than three fourths of patients with the 22Q11.2 deletion have a history of severe or recurrent infection. In these patients, the humoral abnormalities can range from decreased immunoglobulin measurements to abnormal responses to polysaccharide vaccinations. It is recommended that the patients found with 22Q11 deletion should undergo a thorough evaluation of both T-cell function and humoral immunity.

Management

Treatment of patients with complete DiGeorge's syndrome has typically been bone marrow or thymic transplantation.

DiGeorge's Syndrome

- Facial defects, heart defects, hypocalcemia
- Partial DiGeorge's syndrome: low T-cell function
- Complete DiGeorge's syndrome: absent T-cell function
- No spontaneous resolution with complete DiGeorge's syndrome

---

Hyper-IgE Syndrome (Job's Syndrome)

Epidemiology and Etiology

Hyper-IgE syndrome is a multisystem disorder characterized by recurrent skin abscesses, pneumonia with pneumatocele formation, and elevated levels of serum IgE. A genetic linkage to chromosome 4Q has been reported.

Presentation

Patients present with papular, pustular eruptions of the scalp and face in the first year of life; these patients often have persistent eosinophilia. Skin biopsy of the pustules reveals a perivascular dermatitis or folliculitis with a predominance of eosinophils.

Diagnosis

The development of a high IgE level (usually greater than 2,000 μm/mL) and subsequent skin abscesses and/or pneumatoceles, suggest the diagnosis. IgE levels may fluctuate unrelated to the severity of skin disease and infection, and it may be necessary to obtain multiple levels to diagnose the illness. Osteopenia and bone fractures have also been suggested as strongly supportive of the disease. Coarse facial features, as well as delayed loss of primary teeth, is well described in Job's syndrome.

Management

Treatment is supportive, consisting of often long-term treatment with an anti-staphylococcal antibiotic. Surgery may be necessary for persistent pneumatocele formation.

Hyper IgE Syndrome (Job's Syndrome)

- Recurrent skin abscesses
- Papulopustular rashes
- Eosinophilia
- Osteopenia, bone fractures
- Recurrent pneumonia, pneumotocele formation
- IgE levels may fluctuate over time

Chronic Granulomatous Disease

Epidemiology and Etiology

In chronic granulomatous disease (CGD), usually X-linked recessive, patients lack the ability for neutrophil oxidative metabolism. Neutrophils in patients with chronic granulomatous disease cannot produce hydrogen peroxide, which leads to an inability to kill ingested organisms.

Presentation

The most common organism causing infection in patients with CGD is *S. aureus*. Chronic pneumonia progressing to pneumatocele formation is a common presenting sign. CGD may also present with fever of unknown origin and *S. aureus* liver abscesses. *Serratia marcescens* adenitis and sepsis is another typical infection in patients with this condition. *Pseudomonas cepacia*, a common pathogen in end-stage cystic fibrosis, is also seen as a cause of acute and chronic pneumonia in patients with this disorder. Granuloma formation can cause obstruction of the urinary tract; patients present with abdominal pain and hydronephrosis.

Diagnosis

The diagnosis is made by the nitroblue tetrazolium (NBT) test. This test measures oxidative activity in white cells. A normal person will have a test result of 95% to 100%; patients with CGD have a 0% NBT test. In addition to NBT tests, reference laboratories can do genetic analysis to determine the exact genetic mutation and thus the mode of inheritance.

Management

Treatment of patients with CGD includes lifelong prophylaxis against infection. Oral trimethoprim-sulfamethoxazole, as well as itraconazole, is given. These medications decrease the incidence of *S. aureus* and *Aspergillus* species infections, respectively. In addition, subcutaneous gamma interferon (Actimmune), given three times per week, is used as a prophylactic agent. Corticosteroids can be useful in treatment of granulomas causing obstructive symptoms.

Chronic Granulomatous Disease

- Majority are X-linked recessive
- NBT = 0%
- Common infections:
    - *S. aureus*, pneumonia, liver abscess
    - *Aspergillus* species, pneumonia, osteomyelitis
    - *Pseudomonas cepacia*, pneumonia
    - *Serratia marcescens*, adenitis, sepsis

Wiskott-Aldrich Syndrome

Epidemiology and Etiology

Wiskott-Aldrich syndrome is an X-linked disorder that usually becomes symptomatic in early infancy. The responsible gene (*WASP*) has been localized to the X chromosome. Mutations of the gene are thought to affect T-cell functioning. The classic clinical triad of Wiskott-Aldrich is thrombocytopenia, recurrent infections, and eczema.

Presentation

A common presenting sign in patients with this disorder is bleeding following circumcision. Recurrent otitis media and respiratory infections are often seen. Patients can also have abnormalities of both B-cell and T-cell immunity as well as decreased responses to polysaccharide antigens. Children with this condition have elevated IgA and IgE levels accompanied by low levels of IgM.

Diagnosis

The diagnosis is confirmed by the finding of small platelets. Patients with Wiskott-Aldrich syndrome also have an increased incidence of autoimmune disease and malignancies, particularly lymphomas. Prophylactic immunoglobulin and aggressive management of breakthrough bacterial infections is often needed.

Management

Bone marrow transplantation can be curative.

Wiskott-Aldrich Syndrome

- Triad of thrombocytopenia, recurrent infection, and eczema
- Elevated IgA, IgE; decreased IgM
- Small platelets

Common Variable Immunodeficiency

Epidemiology and Etiology

Common variable immunodeficiency (CVI) is similar to Bruton's hypogamma-globulinemia except that it appears to be acquired later in life rather than being present at birth. Patients with CVI do not have the defects in the CD40 ligand or the *BTK* gene mutations that define hyper-IgM and Bruton's agammaglobulinemia syndromes.

The reason certain children lose the ability to make immunoglobulin is not clear. It is possible that this is caused by a variety of conditions rather than a single genetic defect. Patients with CVI may have normal or mildly decreased number of B cells.

Presentation

The clinical manifestations of CVI are similar to those of primary hypogammaglob-ulinemia. Patients have recurrent sinopulmonary disease, often with *H. influenzae* and *S. pneumoniae*. Involvement of the gastrointestinal tract can be seen in patients with CVI; patients may have chronic malabsorption or chronic infection with *Giardia lamblia*. Autoimmune disorders are more frequent in these patients and may include rheumatoid arthritis, systemic lupus erythematosus, and dermatomyositis. The risk for gastric carcinoma and lymphoma is also greatly increased in this population.

Diagnosis

The diagnosis is suggested in a patient who suddenly develops recurrent sinopul-monary infections, often requiring hospitalization and prolonged antibiotics. Immu-noglobulin levels are often markedly decreased, with IgG concentrations less than 300 mg/dL.

Management

Patients need monthly immunoglobulin, usually at a dose of 400 mg/kg. Pneumonia should be aggressively treated, often with long-term broad-spectrum antibiotics. The development of bronchiectasis and chronic lung disease can occur without aggressive and prolonged treatment.

Severe Combined Immunodeficiency

Severe combined immunodeficiency (SCIDS) is a term given to a group of heterogenous disorders characterized by marked deficiency of both B-cell and T-cell immunity.

Epidemiology and Etiology

A large number of genetic defects may result in the final clinical picture of T-cell and B-cell immunodeficiency.

Presentation

Patients are usually ill in the first months of life with failure to thrive and chronic thrush. Severe lymphopenia, interstitial pneumonitis, and PCP are common. Graft-versus-host disease (GVHD) is often seen and represents the "reverse" of the more common host-versus-graft syndrome, in which a recipient (host) rejects a transplanted donor organ (graft). In GVHD, it is usually maternal T cells (graft) present in the neonatal circulation that, in the setting of severe immunodeficiency, attack the child (host).

Diagnosis

Chronic dermatitis represents a common manifestation of GVHD in SCID and should be considered an important clue in the correct clinical setting. Serum levels of all immunoglobulins are usually markedly reduced. Peripheral T-cell number and function are also low. Numerous defined genetic mutations have been shown to result in SCID. In some instances, the genetic basis for the syndrome is unknown.

Management

Therapy is IVIG replacement, prophylactic antibiotics, and consideration for bone marrow transplantation. Early consideration of SCID in the appropriate clinical context is critical because bone marrow transplantation is most successful if done in the first 3 months of life.

Patients with severe combined immunodeficiency must not receive live viral vaccines and should only receive irradiated, white blood cell–depleted blood products.

Severe Combined Immunodeficiency

- Heterogenous causes that result in a deficiency of T-cell and B-cell immunity
- Failure to thrive
- Chronic diarrhea
- GVHD (rashes)
- *Pneumocystis jiroveci* pneumonia

Transient Hypogammaglobulinemia of Infancy

Epidemiology and Etiology

Following birth, maternally derived immunoglobulin declines, with the lowest level reached at about 4 months of age. It is believed that there is a group of infants in whom this physiologic nadir extends beyond 6 months of age. This condition has been termed transient hypogammaglobulinemia of infancy. These children have normal B-cell numbers and normal antibody responses to immunization.

Presentation

Children who have the diagnosis of transient hypogammaglobulinemia of infancy typically have an increased incidence of sinopulmonary infections, such as otitis media, bronchitis, and sinusitis. Infections that are severe or with opportunistic organisms, such as *P. jiroveci*, are unusual and if present should warrant further investigation for an alternative diagnosis.

Diagnosis

It has been suggested that the diagnosis of transient hypogammaglobulinemia can only be made retrospectively. Alternative designations have been proposed, including "hypogammaglobulinemia of early childhood," in which the addition of "recovery" or the "development of dysgammaglobulinemia" can eventually be added. Prospective series of patients with the diagnosis of transient hypogammaglobulinemia of infancy have shown that most children recover with normal immunoglobulin levels by 3 years of age. A minority of patients with transient hypogammaglobulinemia of infancy continue to have low immunoglobulin levels after this time.

Management

Treatment for this condition is generally supportive with aggressive antibiotic therapy for respiratory infections. Immunoglobulin replacement therapy is usually not given. Patients usually outgrow this condition by 2 to 3 years of age, even if measured immunoglobulin concentration has not achieved normal levels.

Transient Hypogammaglobulinemia of Infancy

- Prolonged nadir of immunoglobulin levels following the disappearance of maternal IgG
- Recurrent mild respiratory infections
- Normal B-cell numbers, response to immunizations

IgA Deficiency

Epidemiology and Etiology

Selective IgA deficiency is the most common primary immunodeficiency disease. It is estimated that this immunodeficiency occurs in about in 1 in 500 children in the general population. Patients with this disorder have serum IgA levels of less than 5 mg/dL.

Presentation

Some affected individuals go through life without any difficulty, whereas others have increased numbers of upper respiratory infections. Patients can present with chronic otitis media, sinusitis, or pneumonia. It is thought that patients who have IgA deficiency and chronic respiratory infections may also have associated IgG subclass deficiency.

There are other associations with this disorder, including chronic *Giardia* species infection, autoimmune and rheumatic diseases including inflammatory bowel disease, celiac disease, and systemic lupus erythematosus.

Diagnosis

There is no consensus on when a child with recurrent otitis or sinusitis should have IgA and possibly IgG subclass levels evaluated. Many investigators consider greater than six episodes of otitis media a year a reasonable cutoff for evaluation.

Management

Commercial immunoglobulin preparations do not contain large amounts of IgA. In addition, there is an increased incidence of anaphylactic reactions to immunoglobulin and blood products in patients with IgA deficiency.

Treatment of selective IgA deficiency is **not** monthly IVIG but rather aggressive treatment with antibiotics for respiratory infections.

COMPLEMENT DEFICIENCIES

The classic and alternative complement pathways are initiated by antigen–antibody complexes. Patients with congenital deficiencies of parts of their complement system can be susceptible to infection with a variety of bacteria. The most frequently discussed complement deficiency in pediatrics is terminal portion complement deficiency of C5, C6, C7, C8 or C9.

Terminal Complement Deficiency C5 through C9

Terminal complement deficiency C5 through C9 is associated with increased susceptibility to *Neisseria* species infection.

Epidemiolo gy and Etiology

The terminal complement components C5 to C9 are considered vital in the complement-dependent killing of *Neisseria meningitidis.*

Presentation

There have been estimates that about one half of affected children will develop meningococcal disease. Additional studies have suggested that about 15% of children presenting with their first episode of meningococcal disease have terminal complement deficiency. Some specialists point out that the actual incidence of complement deficiency diagnosed after meningococcal sepsis is highly variable and related to the nationality of the population being studied.

Diagnosis

Many clinicians perform a screening test for complement deficiency on all patients with their first systemic meningococcal or gonococcal infection. An appropriate screening test is a total hemolytic complement (CH50) screening assay. Patients with underlying complement deficiency usually have a level of less than 10 EIA units. In such patients, a complete evaluation for individual complement levels should be done.

Management

Patients identified with complement deficiency should be given the quadrivalent meningococcal vaccine because this may reduce the risk for disease. Some patients are given continuous antimicrobial prophylaxis. Affected patients should have careful counseling on the management of all febrile episodes.

SELECTED READINGS

Bastian J, Law S, Vogler L, et al. Prediction of persistent immunodeficiency in the DiGeorge anomaly. *J Pediatr* 1989;115(3):391–396.

Gennery AR, Barge D, O'Sullivan JJ, et al. Antibody deficiency and autoimmunity in 22 q 11.2 deletion syndrome. *Arch Dis Child* 2002;86(6):422–425.

Leggiadro RJ. Systemic meningococcal infection and complement deficiency. *Pediatr Infect Dis J* 2003;22(8):760–761.

Levy J, Espanol-Boren T, Thomas C, et al. Clinical spectrum of x-linked hyper IgM syndrome. *J Pediatr* 1997;131:47–54.

Overturf GD. Indications for the immunological evaluation of patients with meningitis. *Clin Infect Dis* 2003;36(2):189–194.

Shearer WT, Buckley RH, Engler RJ, et al. Practice parameters for the diagnosis and management of immunodeficiency. The Clinical and Laboratory Immunology Committee of the American Academy of Allergy, Asthma and Immunology (CLIC-AAAAI). *Ann Allergy Asthma Immunol* 1996;76(3): 282–294.

Sneller, MC, Strober W, Eisenstein E, et al. NIH conference: new insights into common variable immunodeficiency. *Ann Intern Med* 1993;118(9):720–730.

5

Hepatitis

BASIC CONSIDERATIONS

The term **hepatitis** refers to any inflammation of the liver.

Although there are many causes of hepatitis in childhood, including toxins and metabolic processes, the most common cause is viral infection. The purpose of this chapter is to review the common viruses that cause hepatitis in childhood and discuss appropriate methods of diagnosis.

HEPATITIS A

Epidemiology and Etiology

Hepatitis A is the most common viral etiology of pediatric hepatitis. The mode of transmission is person to person, resulting from fecal contamination of food. Sexual contact and nosocomial transmission have also been documented.

Presentation

Hepatitis A is an RNA virus that usually causes a self-limited illness associated with fever, jaundice, and anorexia. In children younger than 5 years of age, cases are often anicteric and frequently misdiagnosed as gastroenteritis. Rarely, hepatitis A leads to a fulminant disease, which can be fatal. Chronic infection does not occur, although prolonged disease causing relapsing jaundice has been described.

Diagnosis

The diagnosis of hepatitis A is made by serology. Serum immunoglobulin M (IgM) to hepatitis A is usually present at the onset of illness. The presence of hepatitis A IgG without IgM indicates past infection and immunity.

Management

Currently, there is no specific therapy for hepatitis infection. Treatment is supportive.

Hepatitis A: Major Issues

- Oral–fecal transmission
- Often anicteric in young children
- Diagnosis by hepatitis A IgM
- No chronic carrier state

HEPATITIS B

Epidemiology and Etiology

Hepatitis B is transmitted through blood or body fluids. Transmission by the shared use of nonsterile needles or sexual contact is common in adults.

In the practice of pediatrics, hepatitis B is often transmitted from mothers with chronic infection to their infants at the time of delivery.

Presentation

A wide spectrum of clinical presentations is possible, ranging from nonspecific symptoms of gastroenteritis to fulminant fatal hepatitis.

Diagnosis

There is often considerable confusion regarding the interpretation of hepatitis B serology. The hepatitis B virus (HBV), termed the **Dane particle**, is divided into two basic components: the surface and the core. The core itself has two parts: the core antigen and the e antigen. The presence of high levels of hepatitis B e antigen is correlated with increased levels of circulating levels of HBV DNA and is thought to be a marker for disease activity. Patients who develop antibodies to the hepatitis B e antigen often have a reduction in circulating levels of HBV DNA and improvements in their serum aminotransferase levels. During hepatitis B infection, all persons make antibodies to the core antigen. Subsequent production of antibodies to the surface antigen confers immunity. Failure to produce surface antibodies results in the patient being chronically hepatitis B surface antigen positive; the patient is then diagnosed as a chronic carrier of hepatitis B. The diagnosis of acute or recent hepatitis B infection therefore rests on the presence of IgM antibody to the core antigen because this is the antibody response that **all** patients will make regardless of their ultimate carrier status.

Failure to make hepatitis B surface antibody and development of chronic hepatitis B status are related to the age at the time of infection. Perinatally infected children have a 90% chance of developing chronic infection; children who acquire their infection at 1 through 5 years of age have a 20% to 50% chance of developing chronic infection.

Chronic Infection

Chronic hepatitis B infection progresses to cirrhosis in 15% to 20% of cases. Chronic hepatitis B is also associated with a higher incidence of hepatocellular carcinoma. Protocols in adults suggest that chronic carriers of hepatitis B should be screened yearly for hepatocellular carcinoma using ultrasound examinations and serum α-fetoprotein assays.

Prognosis of chronic hepatitis B infection is based on a variety of factors, including alcohol consumption, prolonged replicative phase, persistent e antigen, and the clearance of hepatitis B surface antigen. Various genotypes of hepatitis B may have an increased likelihood of progressing to chronic disease. Ongoing viral replication and inflammation are thought ultimately to increase the incidence of cirrhosis and hepatocellular carcinoma in patients with chronic hepatitis B infection. The goal of therapy is thus suppression of ongoing viral replication and prevention of these end-stage conditions.

Treatment of Chronic Infection

There has been great interest in identifying patients with chronic infection who will possibly benefit from preemptive therapy. A National Institutes of Health Consensus Workshop on the management of hepatitis B recommended that treatment be considered in patients who are hepatitis B surface antigen positive with an accompanying a viral load of greater than 10^5/mL. This number is somewhat arbitrary; the precise DNA level associated with progressive disease is not known. Aminotransferase levels have been shown to be the best noninvasive marker for the presence of chronic active hepatitis, although up to 40% of patients with histologically confirmed chronic active hepatitis have normal aminotransferase levels. Many specialists consider liver biopsy the best method to determine the need for therapy.

Response to therapy is usually defined as undetectable HBV DNA, loss of hepatitis B antigen, and improvement in liver disease as determined by normalization of aminotransferase levels or by biopsy.

Currently, there are two drugs used for the treatment of hepatitis B infection. Interferon-α has been shown to suppress HBV replication in 30% of adults as compared with 10% of controls. The dose for children is 6 million units/m^2 three times weekly, with a maximum of 10 million units. The recommended duration of treatment is 24 weeks for patients who are hepatitis e antigen positive. Long-term follow-up in adults has suggested that the 5-year cumulative rate of hepatitis B e antigen clearance is similar in untreated patients. The main role of interferon-α may be to hasten viral clearance and thus reduce duration of active liver disease. Patients with high pretreatment aminotransferase levels and low baseline HBV DNA levels appear to have the best response to interferon.

Lamivudine is a nucleotide analog that is frequently used in the treatment of human immunodeficiency virus (HIV) infection. There is increasing use of this drug in patients with chronic hepatitis B infection. Treatment with 3 mg/kg per day (up to 100 mg/day) leads to a significantly higher proportion of children losing hepatitis B e antigen as compared with controls. A major concern in treatment of hepatitis B with lamivudine is the development of the YMDD mutation (thyroxine [y], methionine [m], aspartate [D], and aspartate [D]). These mutations replicate less efficiently than wild-type strains; the long-term implications of the development of these resistant strains are not clear.

Hepatitis B: Treatment

1. Consider treatment in patients with a hepatitis B viral load > 10^5/mL, persistently abnormal aminotransferase levels, or inflammation on liver biopsy.
2. Treatment options include lamivudine, 3 mg/kg per day (maximum, 100 mg/day), or interferon-α, 6 million units/m² three times weekly (maximum, 10 million units).

Guidelines for Adoption

As international adoption becomes more common, there will be an increasing number of hepatitis B surface antigen–positive children residing in the United States. The primary mode of transmission is blood and body secretions; household and day care transmission of hepatitis B is rare. Parents and caretakers should be instructed regarding the following:

- Use thick disposable towels to attend to any bleeding wounds.
- Household items, such as toothbrushes and nail clippers, should not be shared.
- Household contacts should all receive the standard hepatitis B vaccination so that they are protected.

Hepatitis B: Major Issues

- Blood or body fluid transmission
- Diagnosis of acute infection: IgM to hepatitis B core antigen
- Persistence of hepatitis B surface antigen denotes chronic infection.
- Chronic infection is associated with cirrhosis (15% to 20%) and hepatocellular carcinoma.

HEPATITIS C

Epidemiology and Etiology

Hepatitis C virus is transmitted in similar fashion to hepatitis B, through exposure to blood and blood products.

Sexual transmission and transmission among family contacts are rare.

Between 2% and 4% of women of childbearing age are antibody positive for hepatitis C. The vertical transmission rate has been reported to be about 5%, although this increases if the mother is also HIV positive. Most studies have not shown a role in transmission based on the method of delivery. Mothers who are infected with hepatitis C virus may breast-feed their children because transmission through breast milk has not been proved. Transmission from a single needle-stick accident is about 1%.

Hepatitis C: Genotypes

Hepatitis C exists with numerous subtypes, labeled **genotypes**. There are six major genotypes that vary in worldwide distribution and have significance in regard to patient management.

Genotypes 1A and 1B are the most common variants seen in the United States, accounting for more than 75% of all infections. Genotype 2 is more common in the Far East, whereas genotype 3 is frequently seen on the Indian subcontinent. Hepatitis C genotype does not appear to affect the rate of progression, although it is a predictor of a response to therapy. Patients with genotype 2 or 3 are more likely to respond to therapy; those with genotypes 1 and 4 are less likely to respond.

Presentation

The clinical presentation of hepatitis C infection is similar to that of hepatitis A or B: acute disease is often mild and maybe asymptomatic. Only 20% of patients with acute infection become jaundiced.

Diagnosis

Most acute hepatitis C infections are associated with few or no symptoms, making clinical diagnosis difficult. The two available antibody assays are the enzyme immunoassay (EIA) and recombinant immunoblot assay (RIBA). These assays are greater than 95% sensitive and specific, although they can be falsely negative early in disease onset. Viral load or polymerase chain reaction (PCR) assays, similar to those used in detecting HIV, have been developed for hepatitis C. Hepatitis C virus can be detected within 1 to 2 weeks after exposure and weeks before abnormalities in liver enzyme tests are seen.

Hepatitis C antibodies cross the placenta and cannot be used for diagnosis in the neonatal period. The evaluation of the hepatitis C–exposed infant is a hepatitis C PCR at 6 to 8 weeks and again at 6 months of age. Because of the persistence of maternal antibodies in exposed infants, evaluation for hepatitis C antibodies should not be performed until the patient is 1 year of age.

Chronic Infection

Like hepatitis B, hepatitis C infection is associated with a chronic state. The chronic infection is defined by detection of hepatitis C virus by PCR in the blood 6 months after infection. About 60% to 85% of patients infected with hepatitis C develop a chronic infection. The proportion of chronically infected patients who develop the sequelae of hepatitis C is not known. Estimates of 2% to 4% of infected children progressing to cirrhosis and hepatocellular carcinoma have been made. Although viral genotype and baseline viral load do not appear to influence the risk for progression, host factors, including older age at time of infection, alcohol consumption, and coinfection with HIV, may play a role.

Treatment of Chronic Infection

There are evolving treatment options for patients with chronic hepatitis C infection. Because many patients with infection do not have progressive disease, there is great interest in defining patients who will most benefit from therapy. Liver enzymes have shown little value in predicting the degree of fibrosis or cirrhosis in a particular patient. Although hepatitis C RNA (viral load) levels are available by PCR, the situation differs from HIV. In the latter, the viral load is a major factor determining progression of disease and is often involved in the decision to initiate treatment. In the case of hepatitis C, viral load levels do not correlate with either the grade or stage of disease on liver biopsy. There are no currently available noninvasive tests that can reliably predict the level of inflammation or fibrosis of hepatitis C.

The decision to initiate treatment at the present time is usually guided by liver biopsy. Liver biopsy results are evaluated in terms of grade and stage. The grade refers to the level of inflammatory activity and is a measure of ongoing disease. The stage of the liver biopsy refers to the degree of fibrosis and is a measure of disease progression. Patients who have a certain grade of inflammation or fibrosis become candidates for treatment.

Pegylated interferon plus oral ribavirin is currently the standard treatment of hepatitis C. Effective treatment, or sustained viral response (SVR), is defined as the absence of detectable hepatitis C RNA 24 weeks after the end of therapy. Early viral response (EVR) is defined as a minimum 2-log decrease in the viral load during the first 12 weeks of treatment. This is considered highly predictive of SVR. Patients who fail to achieve EVR at week 12 have only a small chance of achieving an SVR, and treatment is often not extended beyond 12 weeks in these patients.

Hepatitis C: Major Issues

- Blood, body fluid transmission
- Acute infection diagnosed by enzyme-linked immunosorbent assay (ELISA) and PCR
- Chronic infection in 60%, associated with cirrhosis, hepatocellular carcinoma

---

EPSTEIN-BARR VIRUS

Epidemiology and Etiology

It is estimated that more than one half of people in the United States will develop Epstein-Barr virus (EBV) infection before the age of 21 years.

EBV is a ubiquitous virus that is frequently the cause of infectious mononucleosis.

Presentation

Adolescents and young adults with infectious mononucleosis typically have fever, severe pharyngitis, rash, and mild to moderate hepatitis. Patients with underlying immunodeficiencies can present with a wider spectrum of disease, including disseminated disease and lymphoproliferative disorders.

Epstein-Barr Virus: Diagnosis

1. VCA is first antibody to appear. IgM antibody lasts about 4 weeks.
2. Early antigen (EA) is the second antibody class to appear. EA is usually detectable several months after acute infection.
3. Nuclear antigen (EBNA) appears during recovery and indicates old infection.

Diagnosis

The diagnosis of EBV is also subject to considerable confusion. The monospot test is frequently used to screen for EBV infection. However, children younger than 5 years of age often do not produce the heterophile antibodies measured by this test. EBV-specific serology is often indicated, although interpretation can be difficult.

Acute EBV infection	Recent EBV infection	Past EBV infection
+IgM, VCA	–IgM, VCA	–IgM, VCA
–IgG, VCA	+IgG, VCA	+IgG, VCA
+EA	+EA	–EA
–EBNA	–EBNA	+EBNA

A variety of antigens have been identified in EBV. The presence of IgM and IgG antibodies to specific antigens is used to diagnose acute or past EBV infection. Viral capsid (VCA) antigens are detected in cells undergoing active EBV infection. Anticapsid antibodies appear at the onset of acute infection and persist for life. IgM to viral capsid antigens is the hallmark of acute EBV infection. Early antigens (EA) are a group of proteins that become positive later in acute infection. EBV nuclear antigen (EBNA) antibodies appear during convalescence and persist for life; anti-EBNA titers indicate **old** EBV infection.

Management

Treatment is generally supportive. Patients with extreme tonsillar hypertrophy who are at risk for airway obstruction can be treated with a brief of course of prednisone, usually 1 mg/kg per day for 5 to 7 days. Because of the potential risk for splenic rupture, contact sports such as martial arts or football should be avoided until the patient has recovered.

CYTOMEGALOVIRUS

Epidemiology

Cytomegalovirus (CMV) is a DNA virus that is also ubiquitous and transmitted person to person and through body fluids such as blood, breast milk, and urine.

Presentation

CMV is another herpesvirus infection that causes a variety of clinical syndromes, the most common being an infectious mononucleosis-like syndrome with prolonged fever and hepatitis. The disease is usually self-limited in immunocompetent individuals, although severe illness can be seen in oncology patients, organ transplant recipients, and patients infected with HIV.

Diagnosis

The diagnosis of acute CMV infection can be complex; diagnosis is difficult because of the large number of asymptomatic persons shedding the virus at any given time. IgM antibody is produced with primary infection, yet can also be produced with reactivated infections. PCR technology can be used, although typically this test is used only in patients with underlying immunodeficiencies. In an immunocompetent patient with a mononucleosis-like syndrome and negative studies for EBV, the diagnosis of CMV is often presumed.

Management

In the immunocompetent patient, care is usually supportive. In certain patient populations such as organ transplant recipients and patients with HIV infection, antiviral therapy with ganciclovir is given.

SELECTED READINGS

Conjeevaram HS, Lok AS. Management of chronic hepatitis B. *J Hepatol* 2003;38[Suppl 1]:S90–103.
Lee WM. Hepatitis B virus infection. *N Engl J Med* 1997;337(24):1733–1745.
Lai CL, Dienstag J, Schiff E, et al. Prevalence and clinical correlates of YMDD variants during lamivudine therapy for patients with chronic hepatitis B. *Clin Infect Dis* 2003;36(6):687–696.
Seef CB, Hoofnagle JH. Appendix: National Institute of Health Consensus Development Conference. Management of hepatitis C. *Clin Liver Dis* 2003;7(1):261–287.

6

Otitis Media and Sinusitis

EPIDEMIOLOGY AND ETIOLOGY

> Otitis media is one of the most common diagnoses in pediatrics.

Immaturity of the eustachian tubes, coupled with a viral upper respiratory infection, can lead to stasis, congestion, and ultimately eustachian tube obstruction. Persisting obstruction of the eustachian tube can result in bacteria being aspirated and trapped in the middle ear, producing a suppurative infection. Because of the frequency of upper respiratory infections in childhood, a child in daycare or with many siblings may experience as many as 6 to 12 episodes of otitis media a year.

Presentation

Pain is considered a common feature of otitis media, which may cause disruptions in sleeping or increased irritability. Although only 25% of children with otitis media are febrile, younger children are more likely to have fever than older children.

Diagnosis

The diagnosis of acute otitis media requires several findings to be present. The first is evidence of middle ear effusion demonstrated by pneumatic otoscopy: middle ear effusion associated with acute otitis media shows impaired or absent mobility of the tympanic membrane. The second is evidence of acute inflammation of the tympanic membranes, usually as opacified bulging of the tympanic membrane or the appearance of a distinct purulent fluid level. Serous otitis media, in which the fluid behind the tympanic membrane is clear without accompanying tympanic membrane bulging, is not considered an acute infectious process and does not require treatment.

Management

General Difficulties in Management of Otitis Media

1. There are increasing numbers of oral antibiotics available for the treatment of otitis media, all claiming to be the "best." It should be remembered that most clinical trials evaluating antibiotics for acute otitis media are designed to show the "equivalency" necessary for U.S. Food and Drug Administration (FDA) approval. Most clinical trials do not demonstrate superiority, and because of the relatively small sample size in most clinical studies, antibiotics with limited efficacy can actually appear to be equal to superior drugs.
2. Unlike many infectious diseases, clinical specimens are not routinely collected for culture and sensitivity. The clinician, therefore, needs to examine the tympanic membrane and make a best guess as to the bacteria responsible.
3. There is increasing resistance to *Streptococcus pneumoniae*, the most common pathogen of otitis media. Two mechanisms of resistance have emerged. For *S. pneumoniae*, the most common cause of otitis media, resistance is due to alterations in penicillin-binding proteins. Resistance to *S. pneumoniae* is defined by the minimal inhibitory concentration (MIC) to penicillin and to third-generation cephalosporins. Penicillin nonsusceptibility in the pneumococcus is defined when the MIC to penicillin is greater than 0.1 µg/mL. The overall rate of penicillin nonsusceptibility for pneumococcus is at least 30%. Pneumococcus isolates considered resistant to penicillin usually have MICs greater than or equal to 2.0 µg/mL; these resistant pneumococcal strains have a high likelihood of resistance to many antibacterial agents. For nonmeningeal infections, pneumococcus nonsusceptibility to third-generation cephalosporins is defined as an MIC greater than 2.0 µg/mL.
4. The other two major pathogens of otitis media are *Haemophilus influenzae* and *Moraxella catarrhalis*. For these organisms, resistance is due to β-lactamase formation. Forty percent of *Haemophilus* strains and virtually all *Moraxella* strains produce β-lactamase, making them resistant to amoxicillin.

Antibiotic Therapy for Otitis Media

Although there are only three major pathogens and only two major mechanisms of resistance, there are many oral antibiotics available for treatment of acute otitis media (Table 6.1). Several generalizations can be made about the many oral antibiotics available for the treatment of acute otitis media. It is important to realize that many of the newer, more expensive second- and third-generation cephalosporins actually have reduced activity against the increasing numbers of penicillin-intermediate and penicillin-resistant *S. pneumoniae*.

1. The first-generation cephalosporins (Cephalexin) have little gram-negative coverage and are usually used to treat gram-positive organisms such as *Streptococcus*

TABLE 6.1. *Major Classes of Antibiotics Used to Treat Otitis Media*

Aminopenicillins
Amoxicillin, 40–80 mg/kg/d; q12
Amoxicillin-clavulanate (Augmentin) (600 mg/5 mL), 90 mg/kg/d of amoxicillin component
Cephalosporins
Second generation
Cefaclor (Ceclor), 20–40 mg/kg/d q8h
Cefuroxime axetil (Ceftin), 30 mg/kg/d q12h
Cefprozil (Cefzil), 30 mg/kg/d q12h
Third generation
Ceftibuten (Cedax), 9 mg/kg/d once
Cefixime (Suprax), 8 mg/kg/d q12h or q24h
Cefpodoxime proxetil (Vantin), 10 mg/kg/d q12h or q24h
Cefdinir (Omnicef), 14 mg/kg/d q12h or q24h
Ceftriaxone (Rocephin), 50 mg/d in 1 to 3 doses
Macrolides
Clarithromycin (Biaxin), 15 mg/kg/d q12h
Azithromycin (Zithromax), 10/kg/d × 1 doses; 5 mg/kg/d × 4 doses
Erythromycin sulfisoxazole (Pediazole), 50 mg/d of erythromycin component in 4 divided doses
Trimethoprim-sulfamethoxazole (Bactrim), 8–10 mg/kg/d of the trimethoprim component q12h

pyogenes and *Staphylococcus aureus*. Generally, first-generation cephalosporins are not used in the treatment of acute otitis media.

2. The second-generation cephalosporins have moderate activity against gram-positive infections with increasing activity against gram-negative bacteria such as *M. catarrhalis* and nontypeable *H. influenzae*. Cefaclor is the least potent of these antibiotics and, because of its association with serum sickness, is generally not used. Cefuroxime (Ceftin) is the most potent of these second-generation cephalosporins against penicillin nonsusceptible pneumococcus, although it has the disadvantage of being difficult for children to accept because of poor taste. Cefprozil (Cefzil) is intermediate in both taste and potency.

3. The third-generation cephalosporins have excellent gram-negative activity. However, activity against gram-positive organisms is variable. Cefixime (Suprax) and ceftibuten (Cedax) have reduced efficacy against penicillin non-susceptible *S. pneumoniae* and are poor choices for the treatment of acute otitis media caused by this organism. These agents have good activity against penicillin-sensitive pneumococcus as well as β-lactamase–producing *H. influenzae* and *M. catarrhalis*.

4. The macrolide antibiotics include erythromycin, clarithromycin, and azithromycin. Although these were formerly front-line therapies for sinusitis and acute otitis media, there has been increasing resistance of pneumococcus, group A streptococci, and *H. influenzae* to macrolide antibiotics. Currently, about 30% of all strains of *S. pneumoniae* demonstrate *in vitro* resistance to macrolides. Although the exact relationship of *in vitro* macrolide resistance to actual clinical outcome is not always clear, many specialists believe that these drugs are poor agents for the treatment of upper respiratory infections and should be reserved for use in the management of

lower respiratory infections in children who are likely to have atypical pathogens, such as *Mycoplasma pneumoniae* and *Chlamydia pneumoniae*.
5. Trimethoprim-sulfamethoxazole (Bactrim) was previously a mainstay of therapy for the treatment of sinusitis and acute otitis media. There has been increased resistance of *S. pneumoniae* to trimethoprim-sulfamethoxazole (more than 30%), and it is no longer recommended as front-line therapy.

Treatment Recommendations

In 1999, the Centers for Disease Control and Prevention convened a working group that published recommendations regarding the treatment of acute otitis media. Initial treatment was recommended with amoxicillin at a dose of 80 to 100 mg/kg per day. Amoxicillin given at the previous standard doses of 40 to 45 mg/kg per day was determined not to achieve middle ear fluid levels that would eradicate the increasingly prevalent penicillin nonsusceptible pneumococcal strains. The increase in dosing to 80 to 100 mg/kg per day was thought to achieve higher antibiotic levels in the middle ear and be effective against these strains. This regimen would also be efficacious against *M. catarrhalis* and *H. influenzae* strains that did not produce β-lactamase.

Treatment failures, defined as lack of clinical improvement after 3 days of therapy, would likely be secondary to resistant pneumococcus or β-lactamase–producing *H. influenzae* or *M. catarrhalis*. The panel recommended the following treatment options:

• Cefuroxime axetil (Ceftin)
• Intramuscular ceftriaxone (Rocephin)
• Amoxicillin clavulanate (Augmentin)
• Clindamycin

There was excellent logic to these recommendations. However, it should be remembered that these were guidelines developed at a certain time. The panel did state that, at the time of publication, there was not enough evidence of efficacy for certain drugs against the resistant pneumococcus that may be responsible for most treatment failures. In the subsequent years, the rates of resistance of *S. pneumoniae* have only increased. Additional developments regarding treatment of penicillin-nonsusceptible and penicillin-resistant *S. pneumoniae* also include the following:

1. There remains limited clinical experience using clindamycin, and no consensus exists on the actual number of injections of intramuscular ceftriaxone required for treatment of acute otitis media. Some investigators have found that up to three intramuscular injections are needed for resolution of acute otitis media.
2. New formulations of antibiotics have become available, including high-dose amoxicillin combined with clavulanic acid (Augmentin ES, 600 mg per 5 mL).
3. Experience has increased in the treatment of resistant *S. pneumoniae* with several third-generation oral cephalosporins, such as cefdinir and cefpodoxime.

Recommendations for treatment of otitis media have recently been revised. Amoxicillin remains the initial choice for primary therapy. Children at low risk for infection with penicillin-nonsusceptible *S. pneumoniae* can be treated with 40 mg/kg per day in two divided doses. Even with the *S. pneumoniae* classified as resistant to penicillin, it is thought that high-dose amoxicillin (80 to 90 mg/kg per day) achieves sufficiently high levels in the middle ear to achieve cure. In children with increased risk for infection with penicillin-resistant *S. pneumoniae*, including those younger than 2 years of age, attending daycare, or having received antibiotics within the preceding 30 days, therapy should be started using the high dose of 80 to 90 mg/kg per day in two divided doses.

For children with clinically defined treatment failure at 48 to 72 hours, several antibiotics have been recommended as second-line therapy. Treatment options include the following:

- Amoxicillin clavulanate, using the high-dose formulation of 600 mg per 5 mL, given as 90 mg/kg per day of the amoxicillin component in two divided doses
- Oral therapy with cefdinir, cefuroxime axetil, or cefpodoxime
- Intramuscular ceftriaxone, 50 mg/kg for one to three doses

As resistance patterns change, recommendations will need to be updated.

Treatment Delay

As antibiotic resistance becomes more prevalent, there is continued discussion about treatment delay in otitis media. It has been determined that a significant percentage of acute otitis media resolves in 2 to 7 days without antibiotic therapy. An increasing strategy, particularly in foreign countries, is to withhold treatment in a patient with early otitis media. Children are then rechecked in 48 to 72 hours to determine whether infection has resolved. Delaying treatment does not substantially increase the risk for complications, including the rate of severe mastoiditis.

Surgical Management of Otitis Media

The role of surgical intervention in patients with otitis media, particularly recurrent otitis media, is often debated. There is concern about the effect of recurrent otitis media and persistent middle ear effusions in young children at the age of language development. Various studies have addressed the issue of developmental outcomes in children with persistent otitis media and effusions. Although a variety of conclusions have been drawn, a recent study reported no improvement in the developmental outcomes at 3 years in children who had prompt insertion of tympanostomy tubes by 9 months of life. Tympanostomy tube insertion in children is often still considered if there is chronic effusion lasting 3 months or longer, documented hearing loss, or recurrent otitis media, defined as three or more episodes during the previous 6 months or four or more episodes during the past year.

CHRONIC SUPPURATIVE OTITIS MEDIA

Epidemiology and Etiology

> Chronic ear drainage (otorrhea) is defined as drainage lasting greater than 6 weeks.

The most common cause of chronic ear drainage in pediatrics is chronic suppurative otitis media (CSOM). CSOM is defined as a chronic infection of the middle ear and mastoid associated with a nonintact tympanic membrane or a tympanostomy tube. CSOM may develop following an episode of acute otitis media with perforation and subsequent development of chronic drainage. CSOM may also be caused by a chronic perforation of the tympanic membrane in which the middle ear becomes infected by environmental organisms. The bacteria causing CSOM often differ from those of acute otitis media; the most common organisms involved include *Pseudomonas aeruginosa* and *S. aureus*. Rarely, this condition can be caused by *Candida* species or anaerobic bacteria.

Presentation

Affected children present with a history of ear drainage for many weeks. Typically, these children have had numerous courses of oral antibiotics.

Diagnosis

Diagnosis is usually suggested by the history. Culture of the ear drainage that yields the typical bacteria in the correct clinical context also suggest the diagnosis.

Management

Management of the chronic draining ear can begin on an outpatient basis. Culture of ear drainage can be obtained to document the typical pathogens of CSOM. In the past, a variety of ototopical agents were used. These medications were often ophthalmologic drops, which lacked efficacy against the typical CSOM pathogens and were potentially ototoxic. Ofloxacin is a topical fluoroquinolone that has been approved for use in children with tympanostomy tubes. This is now often considered a front-line ototopical agent when CSOM is diagnosed. In addition to antimicrobial therapy, good aural toilet is necessary. Children may need daily visits to the otolaryngologist for suctioning and installation of appropriate topical agents in the middle ear.

If a patient fails to respond to ototopical therapy, consideration of parental antibiotics may be needed. Because there is no approved oral antimicrobial for treatment of

Pseudomonas species infection in children, hospitalization may be needed for administration of an appropriate intravenous drug such as ceftazidime. Computed tomography may be necessary at this time to document chronic osteomyelitis or a mass lesion.

SINUSITIS

Etiology

Like otitis media, bacterial sinusitis is believed to be the result of a preceding viral upper respiratory infection that predisposes to a secondary bacterial infection.

> Sinusitis is similar to otitis media in that it is a common upper respiratory infection in which the diagnosis is based on clinical parameters rather than isolation of a causal organism.

Presentation

The diagnosis of bacterial sinusitis is based on the history of upper respiratory infection. Children with high fever and purulent nasal discharge for 3 to 4 days should have the diagnosis considered. Children with persistent symptoms that last longer than 10 to 14 days are considered to have a high probability of a bacterial infection.

Diagnosis

The gold standard of the diagnosis of sinusitis is the recovery of more than 10^4 colony forming units/mL from a sinus aspirate, although this procedure will not be routinely employed in the pediatric office. Thus, the diagnosis of bacterial sinusitis is based on clinical criteria. As mentioned earlier, the basis for the clinical diagnosis of sinusitis is the presence of persistent symptoms. An upper respiratory infection that has lasted longer than 10 to 14 days is the best feature distinguishing sinusitis from a routine viral infection. Severe symptoms, defined as a temperature of at least 38.8°C (102°F) with purulent nasal discharge for at least 3 consecutive days, are also acceptable clinical criteria.

The physical examination is not particularly helpful in distinguishing between viral upper respiratory infection and sinusitis. Transillumination of the sinuses has been proposed, although reviews have suggested that this is difficult to perform correctly and is not reliable in young children. Imaging studies are not necessary to establish a diagnosis of sinusitis in children younger than 6 years of age. Plain films and computed tomography of the paranasal studies show mucosal thickening in both viral and bacterial upper respiratory disease. For the general practitioner, the history and duration of symptoms are the basis for an accurate diagnosis of bacterial sinusitis.

Management

The microbiology of acute sinusitis is similar to that of acute otitis media. The principal bacterial pathogens include *S. pneumoniae*, nontypeable *H. influenzae*, and *M. catarrhalis*. The increasing resistance of *S. pneumoniae* to penicillin and the large percentage of *Moraxella* and *Haemophilus* strains that produce β-lactamase also affect the treatment of sinusitis in children. Because organisms and resistance profile are similar, current recommendations for the treatment of otitis media can generally be applied to sinusitis.

SELECTED READINGS

American Academy of Pediatrics. Subcommittee on Management of Sinusitis and Committee on Quality Improvement. Clinical practice guideline: management of sinusitis. *Pediatrics* 2001;108(3)798–808.

Bluestone CD, Klein JO. Chronic suppurative otitis media. *Pediatr Rev* 1999;20(8):277–279.

Bluestone CD. Role of surgery for otitis media in the era of resistant bacteria. *Pediatr Infect Dis J* 1998;17(11):1090–1098.

Faden H, Duffy L, Boeve M. Otitis media: back to basics. *Pediatr Infect Dis J* 1998;17:1105–1112.

Paradise JL, Dollaghan CA, Campbell TF, et al. Otitis media and tympanostomy tube insertion during the first three years of life: developmental outcomes at the age of four years. *Pediatrics* 2003;112(2):265–277.

Rosenfeld RM, Vertrees JE, Carr J, et al. Clinical efficacy of antimicrobial drugs for acute otitis media: meta-analysis of 5,400 children from thirty-three randomized trials. *J Pediatr* 1994;124(3):355–367.

7

Outpatient Evaluation of Fever

BASIC ISSUES IN PEDIATRIC FEVER

Fever is a common presenting complaint in pediatrics. The pediatrician's concern about fever in a child can be summarized by the following questions:

1. What is the chance, given this temperature elevation, that this child has an evolving serious bacterial infection?
2. What should be the proper evaluation and empiric treatment concerning this possibility of an evolving serious bacterial infection?

> These questions relates only to the well-appearing pediatric patient. Children who are toxic, hypotensive, have altered mental status or decreased peripheral perfusion should be managed aggressively regardless of initial laboratory evaluations.

The question regarding the management of the well-appearing, nontoxic, febrile infant remains one of the most controversial in pediatrics and emergency medicine. Proposed strategies are constantly revised and depend on the child's age, underlying condition of the child, and development of new vaccinations. One traditional approach is to divide the evaluation of the febrile child by age.

NEONATE (0 TO 28 DAYS)

Epidemiology and Etiology

More than one half of all women have bacterial genital tract colonization, often with group B streptococcus. About one half of neonates born to colonized women themselves become colonized. Of these colonized infants, about 1% develop invasive disease. Risk factors for invasive neonatal disease include prematurity, maternal fever during delivery, and prolonged rupture of membranes.

There are certain patient populations in which the chance of a serious bacterial infection is high and the physical exam and laboratory evaluations nonspecific enough that a full workup and empiric antibiotics are always indicated. Such a patient is the child in the first month of life.

Presentation

> Neonates with rectal temperatures greater than 38°C (100.4°F) have an overall risk of 13% for serious bacterial infection.

The history, physical exam, and even complete laboratory evaluations do not separate these infants into "high-risk" (high statistical likelihood to have a serious bacterial infection) and "low-risk" categories.

Diagnosis

Studies have suggested that even a negative full diagnostic workup, including complete blood count, urinalysis, stool Gram stain, and lumbar puncture, will miss a percentage of neonates who ultimately have a serious bacterial infection, including bacteremia and urinary tract infections.

Management

Two regimens are accepted for empiric treatment of neonatal fever. Ampicillin is usually given to address the possibility of *Listeria monocytogenes* infection. The second agent given is usually a third-generation cephalosporin or gentamycin to cover gram-negative organisms.

Standard practice continues to be a full evaluation and admission for intravenous antibiotics pending results of blood, urine, and cerebrospinal fluid (CSF) cultures.

INFANT (28 TO 59 DAYS)

For the child older than 1 month of age, efforts begin to define those children whose risk for a serious bacterial infection is such that they could be managed as outpatients and avoid the automatic admission with intravenous antibiotics.

Etiology

The organisms in this population are similar to those found in the neonatal group, with group B streptococcus, gram-negative enteric organisms and occasionally *Streptococcus pneumoniae* being the major pathogens.

Presentation

Definition of fever in this population is similar to that in the neonatal group.

Diagnosis

In the early 1980s, the first attempt was made to develop diagnostic criteria. The Yale Observation Scale was entirely clinical and measured characteristics such as cry, social response, and hydration status. This was found to have a negative predictive value of about 80%; that is, up to 20% of those who satisfied criteria for discharge did indeed have a serious bacterial infection. This rate was not sensitive enough to satisfy most clinicians.

The Rochester Criteria in the late 1980s was the first to attempt to incorporate laboratory data in evaluation of the febrile infant. The Rochester Criteria used white blood cell (WBC) count, urinalysis, and stool WBC count as part of the protocol. Major criticisms of these criteria were that CSF analysis was not included and that the criteria did not include clinical impression as part of the evaluation process.

Next came the Baskin Study in 1992. In this protocol, infants 1 to 2 months of age with a rectal temperature of greater than 38°C (100.4°F) and a nontoxic appearance received a full laboratory evaluation, including lumbar puncture, complete blood count, urinalysis, and stool studies. Patients with unremarkable findings on these screening tests received intramuscular ceftriaxone before discharge with close follow-up. Although there were a number of positive blood, urine, and stool cultures, these children had negative cultures on follow-up evaluation, and no complications were noted as a result of outpatient management. Criticisms of the study included the use of a dipstick urine evaluation rather than a microscopic urinalysis and, most importantly, no control population. It was thought that this protocol essentially substituted intravenous antibiotic therapy with outpatient intramuscular ceftriaxone.

In 1993, Baker and colleagues developed the Philadelphia Protocol. In this study, febrile infants between 1 and 2 months of age all received a full diagnostic workup including lumbar puncture, urinalysis, and stool studies if diarrhea was present. A low-risk infant was defined as having a peripheral WBC count of less than 15,000/mm^3, less than 10 WBCs per high-power field on urinalysis, a CSF with less than 8 WBCs per high-power field, and no evidence of a focal soft tissue infection. The criteria also included a peripheral blood band–to-neutrophil ratio of less than 0.2. These screening criteria were found to be 100% sensitive in identifying those children with serious bacterial illnesses, with a negative predictive value of 100%. Patients who had negative diagnostic evaluations were actually discharged home with no antibiotic therapy given. The negative predictive value was such that this study is cited today as proof that a select group of infants between the ages of 1 and 2 months can be managed as outpatients without intravenous or intramuscular antibiotics.

Management

It has been suggested that no plan for outpatient management of febrile children in this age group is entirely without risk. Guidelines continue to be revised and new recommendations formulated, including those that give the option of deferring lumbar puncture in the correct low-risk setting.

The C-reactive protein (CRP) is an acute-phase reactant that is sometimes used as an indicator for evolving serious bacterial infections. Some studies have found the CRP to be a better indicator than the peripheral WBC count or absolute neutrophil count in predicting those febrile infants who truly have an evolving bacterial infection. A CRP of less than 5 mg/dL has been cited as the cutoff for effectively ruling out bacterial infection. Some investigators have suggested that a lumbar puncture can be deferred if the CRP is less than 5 mg/dL. Recent guidelines by Baraff and associates (2000) suggest that if lumbar puncture is deferred, empiric antibiotics should not be given because pretreatment of a child in whom the CSF has not been examined may make subsequent interpretation of the CSF difficult.

Low-Risk Criteria for Febrile Infants (30 to 59 days)

- Serum WBCs: 5 to 15,000/m^3, <1,500 bands/m^3
- Urinalysis: <10 WBCs/high-power field
- When diarrhea present, <5 WBC/high-power field in stool
- CSF: <8 WBC/high-power field, negative Gram stain
- CRP: <5 mg/dL

Recent guidelines have suggested the following options: all febrile infants receive a complete blood count, urinalysis, CRP, and blood and urine culture. Options outlined in Table 7.1.

TABLE 7.1. *Management of the Nontoxic Febrile Infants, 28 to 59 Days of Age*

Option 1
a. "Low-risk" infant
b. Lumbar puncture obtained; consider no treatment or 50 mg/kg of intramuscular ceftriaxone
c. Close follow-up
Option 2
a. "Low-risk" infant
b. C-reactive protein < 5 mg/dL, lumbar puncture deferred, antibiotics not given
c. Close follow-up
Option 3
a. "High-risk" infant
b. C-reactive protein > 5 mg/dL, lumbar puncture required
c. Consider hospital admission, empiric antibiotics

CHILDREN (3 MONTHS TO 36 MONTHS)

Epidemiology and Etiology

As in the case of the well-appearing febrile infant, there remains considerable debate about management of a febrile child aged 3 months to 3 years.

In the early 1970s, the first reports appeared of *S. pneumoniae* bacteremia in well-appearing febrile children. The reported rate of bacteremia in febrile, well-appearing children was approximately 4% and was labeled "benign" because most of these children had resolution of bacteremia without sequelae. After these early reports, numerous studies attempted to determine the actual morbidity associated with this "silent" bacteremia in children. The concern is that this bacteremia could result in one of the following:

- Persistent fever
- Progression to sepsis, especially in the case of *Neisseria meningitidis* (Fig. 7.1)
- "Seeding" of secondary sites; the most feared site being the CSF (Fig. 7.2)

The widespread use of *H. influenzae* conjugate vaccine has essentially eliminated this pathogen. The organism currently causing 90% of the bacteremia in this age group is *S. pneumoniae*. Bacteria less frequently encountered include *Salmonella* species and *N. meningitidis*.

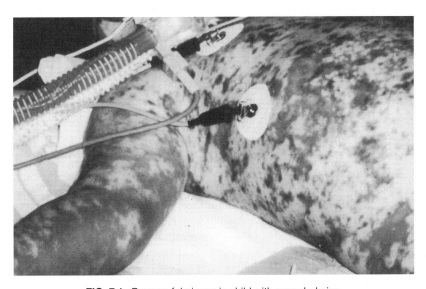

FIG. 7.1. Purpura fulminans in child with overwhelming
Neisseria meningitidis infection (see color plate).

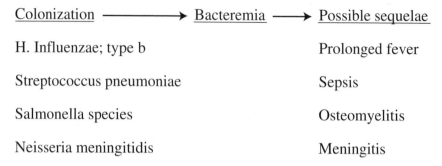

Colonization ⟶ Bacteremia ⟶ Possible sequelae

H. Influenzae; type b	Prolonged fever
Streptococcus pneumoniae	Sepsis
Salmonella species	Osteomyelitis
Neisseria meningitidis	Meningitis

FIG. 7.2. Mechanism and potential sequelae of pediatric bacteremia.

Presentation

Children with pneumococcal bacteremia often present with sudden onset of high fever. There are typically nontoxic in appearance, and no focus is found on physical examination.

Diagnosis

About 2% to 3% of febrile children are bacteremic. In addition, about 3% of these bacteremia patients may progress to meningitis. Thus, the basic questions confronting the clinician while examining a well-appearing febrile child with no focus of infection are the following:

1. How do we identify those children who are actually bacteremic at the time of evaluation?
2. Does presumptive treatment in these children with either oral or intramuscular antibiotics actually alter the natural history of the bacteremia? Although it makes theoretical sense that bacteremic children identified early and presumptively treated have reduced progression to complications of bacteremia (i.e., meningitis), is this indeed the case?

Management

In 1993, Baraff published guidelines for the management of fever in children. In this publication, it was suggested that when evaluating fever without a source in children, a complete blood count should be obtained. If the WBC count was more than 15,000/mm^3, this represented an increased chance of bacteremia with the resultant chance (albeit small) of meningitis. It has been recommended to give antibiotic treatment to these children to prevent the chance of meningitis.

Baraff's guidelines were offered as suggestions, yet rapidly became the standard of care. Infants with fever without a source routinely had complete blood counts and blood cultures obtained and empiric antibiotics given. The concern was that this abundance of antibiotics would generate increased bacterial resistance (a concern that has proved correct). In addition, there was no conclusive evidence that empiric antibiotics truly prevented the bacteremia progressing to meningitis. Over the next 10 years, many studies sought to address the issue of empiric treatment. The methodology and results of these studies continue to be debated.

In 1994, Fleisher and associates performed a multicenter study of more than 6,000 children. In this study, children 3 to 36 months of age with a temperature of more than 39°C (102.2°F) had a blood culture obtained and were given either a single dose of ceftriaxone or oral amoxicillin. The incidence of bacteremia was 2.8%. In the analysis of the data, the authors stated that fewer children who were treated with ceftriaxone developed meningitis than those who were given oral amoxicillin. This study continues to be frequently quoted as evidence that antibiotics given to febrile children will prevent meningitis.

In an accompanying editorial, Dr. Sara Long (1994) both praised the study and commented on its shortcomings. She commented that less than one fourth of all febrile children had examinations of the CSF. One of the patients with meningitis placed to the amoxicillin group actually had pneumococcus isolated from the CSF before therapy was begun; Dr. Long commented that this should have been reported as a misdiagnosis, not amoxicillin failure. Two of the ceftriaxone-treated children with bacteremia caused by *H. influenzae* type B and *Salmonella* species had, on repeat visit, a CSF pleocytosis of 117 and 158 WBCs, respectively. Although this did not meet the preset requirements of more than 500 WBCs for the diagnosis of meningitis, Dr. Long suggested that most infectious disease specialists would indeed consider these two cases, in a setting of prior bacteremia, to be bacterial meningitis that had developed despite the administration of ceftriaxone. Dr. Long concluded that there were still no data that ceftriaxone, or any antibiotic, prevented the rare occurrence of pneumococcal meningitis.

In 1997, Rothrock and colleagues undertook a meta-analysis of several published studies to determine whether oral antibiotics given to febrile children prevented serious bacterial infections or meningitis in patients with *S. pneumoniae* bacteremia. Ten available studies with 656 total cases of *S. pneumoniae* occult bacteremia were identified. Patients who received oral antibiotics had fewer serious bacterial infections than untreated patients, 3.3% versus 9.7%. Meningitis developed in 0.8% of children in the oral antibiotic group and 2.7% of untreated children. The authors themselves concluded that the modest decreased risk for serious bacterial infection in patients with occult pneumococcal bacteremia was "insufficient evidence" to state that oral antibiotics prevented meningitis. Subsequent reviewers, citing this article, have pointed to the reduced number of cases of meningitis as proof that antibiotics were effective and warranted.

In 2000, Alpern and associates retrospectively reviewed 5,900 children 2 to 24 months of age with temperature higher than 39°C (102.2°F). Patients with positive cultures for pathogenic bacteria were evaluated and their outcomes determined. Occult bacteremia was seen in 1.9%. Ninety-six percent of patients with pneumococcal bacteremia had resolution of their bacteremia without the use of parental antibiotics. The rate of meningitis or death was 0.03%. These numbers were significantly less than the rates of bacteremia and meningitis determined in prior studies. The authors concluded that the conjugate *Haemophilus* vaccine and the ability to monitor blood cultures continuously, which allows for early detection of bacteremia, resulted in low rates of adverse outcomes from occult bacteremia. The authors suggested that these findings should be considered in management strategies. They also stated that the development of a conjugate vaccine against *S. pneumoniae* may "ultimately lay the issue to rest."

In December 2000, in anticipation of the approval of the conjugate pneumococcal vaccine, Baraff published revised guidelines for the management of fever without a source in infants and children. The author noted that the anticipated widespread use of conjugate pneumococcal vaccine might very well make the use of WBC count and blood cultures, with empiric antibiotic treatment becoming obsolete.

Baraff recommended raising the temperature threshold for obtaining screening WBC to 39.5°C (103.1°F). He also suggested the following strategy:

1. In patients 3 years of age and older, no testing is required for temperatures lower than 39°C (102.2°F) because the risk for bacteremia is less than 1%.
2. Complete blood counts and blood cultures should be obtained in children younger than 3 years of age with fever without a source and a temperature higher than 39.5°C (103.1°F). Patients who have fever without a source who are 3 to 24 months of age with a temperature higher than 39°C (102.2°F) should also have these tests because the risk for bacteremia in this age group is about 3%.
3. Urinalysis and urine culture should be obtained in all febrile males 6 months of age and younger and in uncircumcised males 6 to 12 months of age. All females younger than 12 months of age should also receive urinalysis and culture.
4. In patients whose WBC count is more than 15,000/m³ or whose absolute neutrophil count is more than 10,000 mm³, the risk for pneumococcal bacteremia is about 8%. In these patients, the administration of empiric antibiotics could be considered. Ceftriaxone has been recommended, although many practitioners will continue to use oral amoxicillin.

FUTURE CONSIDERATIONS

Management strategies are not intended to be rigidly applied in every circumstance. Physicians have the option to tailor their management on the basis of such factors as follow-up, the presence of a telephone, and the ability of a patient to return for reevaluation the following day. Emergency room physicians often treat more aggressively than a private practice pediatrician who knows that he or she will be able to speak with the family in 6 hours. In the era of conjugate vaccines for both *H. influenzae* and *S. pneumoniae*, there continues to be a turn away from rigid protocols involving complete blood cell counts, blood cultures, and empiric treatment.

Many physicians currently advocate a "no test, no treatment" strategy with careful watchful waiting, as was done in the early 1970s before the beginning of the "bacteremia bandwagon." As the incidence of bacteremia decreases, the emphasis may be more on observation and close follow-up than on laboratory evaluation and empiric therapy.

SELECTED READINGS

Alpern ER, Alessandrini EA, Bell LM, et al. Occult bacteremia from a pediatric emergency department: current prevalence, time to detection, and outcome. *Pediatrics* 2000;106(3):505–511.

Baker MD, Bell LM, Avner JR. The efficacy of routine outpatient management without antibiotics of fever in selected Infants. *Pediatrics* 1999;103(3):627–631.

Baraff LJ. Management of fever without source in infants and children. *Ann Emerg Med* 2000;36(6): 602–614.

Fleisher GR, Rosenberg N, Vinci R, et al. Intramuscular versus oral antibiotic therapy for the prevention of meningitis and other bacterial sequelae in young, febrile children at risk for occult bacteremia. *J Pediatr* 1994;124(4):504–512.

Issacman DJ, Burke BL. Utility of the serum c-reactive protein for detection of occult bacterial infection in children. *Arch Pediatr Adolesc Med* 2002;156(9):905–909.

Long SS. Antibiotic therapy in febrile children: "best laid schemes." *J Pediatr* 1994;124(4):585–588.

Roth Rock SG, Green SM, Harper MB, et al. Parental vs. oral antibiotics in the prevention of serious bacterial infections in children with *Streptococcus pneumoniae* occult bacteremia: a meta-analysis. *Acad Emerg Med* 1998;5(6)599–606.

8

Periorbital and Orbital Cellulitis

The red, swollen eye is a common presenting symptom in pediatrics. As is the case for many pediatric infections, there are three mechanisms of disease for the red eye. Each of these mechanisms involves different presenting symptoms, different causative pathogens, and different management strategies.

MECHANISM OF DIRECT INOCULATION

This process involves introduction of a pathogen into the eye or the soft tissue surrounding the eye. In the former, one develops viral or bacterial conjunctivitis. In the latter case, one develops a periorbital cellulitis.

Ophthalmia Neonatorum

Epidemiology and Etiology

Ophthalmia neonatorum is defined as conjunctivitis in the first weeks of life. *Neisseria gonorrhoeae* and *Chlamydia trachomatis* infections are the most common causes of neonatal conjunctivitis. *N. gonorrhoeae* infection in the newborn infant typically involves the eyes and is caused by exposure at the time of delivery.

Chlamydia trachomatis is the other major pathogen of neonatal conjunctivitis. As with gonococcal disease, exposure is at the time of delivery. The risk for conjunctivitis to a baby who is exposed is about 50%, with 20% of exposed infants eventually developing pneumonia.

Presentation

Neonates usually present during the first weeks of life with a purulent conjunctivitis. Disease attributable to *C. trachomatis* is often not as severe as that caused by *N. gonorrhoeae* and may present later in the neonatal period.

Diagnosis

Gram stain of the conjunctival discharge may reveal gram-negative diplococci. Newborns with *N. gonorrhoeae* disease should have cultures of blood and spinal fluid because disseminated disease can occur.

Neonatal *C. trachomatis* conjunctivitis can be diagnosed by the appearance of intracytoplasmic inclusions on Giemsa stain of conjunctival scrapings. There is considerable variation in the sensitivity of this test up to 90%, depending on collection technique and laboratory experience with conjunctival specimens. Direct fluorescent antibody and polymerase chain reaction testing for *Chlamydia* antigen are also used on conjunctival scrapings in patients suspected of having *C. trachomatis* infection.

Management

Ceftriaxone is the therapy of choice for gonococcal infections because an increasing number of isolates are showing resistance to penicillin. Infants with gonococcal conjunctivitis need frequent eye irrigation because the purulent discharge is very damaging to the cornea and can result in permanent scarring.

Chlamydia trachomatis

Treatment of infants with *C. trachomatis* conjunctivitis is always with oral erythromycin, 50 mg/kg per day in four divided doses for 2 weeks. Topical treatment of *C. trachomatis* conjunctivitis is not recommended; systemic treatment is needed to prevent subsequent development of lower respiratory tract disease.

For newborns diagnosed with either gonococcal or chlamydial conjunctivitis, evaluation for other sexually transmitted diseases, including syphilis, hepatitis B, hepatitis C, and human immunodeficiency virus (HIV) infection, should be considered.

Conjunctivitis in Toddlers

Epidemiology and Etiology

The etiologic agents of pediatric conjunctivitis were investigated for the first time in the 1980s. About 80% of cases were found to be bacterial in origin. Nontypeable *Haemophilus influenzae* was recovered in almost half of cases; *Streptococcus pneumoniae* was the other common bacterial agent. Adenovirus was the most common viral pathogen isolated.

Presentation

Distinguishing viral from bacterial conjunctivitis clinically can be difficult. Bacterial conjunctivitis typically affects children younger than 5 years of age. Children present with a purulent discharge that often causes the eyelids to be stuck together after a night's sleep. Adenoviral conjunctivitis often occurs in the fall and winter and usually in children older than 6 years of age. It can be associated with sore throat and low-grade fever. Adenovirus is very contagious, and epidemics involving athletic groups or persons with common exposure to water or fomites are well described. Adenovirus conjunctivitis can also cause a symptom that may mimic a bacterial periorbital infection. Although older children with adenovirus conjunctivitis may have minimal eyelid swelling, younger children may exhibit considerable edema and swelling that can appear very similar to bacterial periorbital cellulitis.

Diagnosis

Reviews have noted that an inflammatory membrane on the conjunctiva is a consistent physical finding for adenovirus conjunctivitis and can be helpful in the diagnosis.

An additional concern is that acute adenoviral conjunctivitis, with its associated fever and pharyngitis, may mimic Kawasaki syndrome. Studies have shown that children with acute adenoviral infection are likely to have purulent conjunctivitis, lower levels of alanine amino transferase, and lower sedimentation rates. A rapid antigen test for adenovirus done on a conjunctival swab can be helpful in distinguishing adenoviral conjunctivitis from Kawasaki syndrome.

Management

Pediatricians often empirically treat conjunctivitis with antibacterial agents. This approach seems reasonable, given the high incidence of bacteria causing acute conjunctivitis. Attempts to have formal laboratory diagnosis can include obtaining Gram stain and culture of the purulent discharge or conjunctival scrapings. It has been found that Gram stain and cultures of conjunctival scrapings obtained by ophthalmologists have a higher yield than cultures of conjunctival exudate. Most pediatricians are not experienced in obtaining conjunctival scrapings, although Gram stain of conjunctival exudate showing more than 15 white blood cells per high-power field may be helpful in distinguishing bacterial from viral conjunctivitis.

Although acute bacterial conjunctivitis is known to be a self-limited disease, double-blind placebo-controlled studies have shown that treatment with either topical or oral antibiotics resulted in earlier clinical improvement and earlier eradication of bacteria from the conjunctivae. It is for this reason that bacterial conjunctivitis is usually treated.

There are a variety of topical antibiotics available, including trimethoprim, polymyxin B, gentamycin sulfate, and sodium sulfacetamide. Also now available are the topical fluoroquinolones, approved for children older than 1 year. It has been suggested in the past that if first-line topical therapy for acute conjunctivitis is not successful, one should consider obtaining a culture and consider using a topical fluoroquinolone to address the possibility of a resistant pathogen. A recent report measured increasing antibiotic resistance in bacteria isolated from children with bacterial conjunctivitis; β-lactamase production was detected in almost 70% of strains of *H. influenzae*; over one third of *S. pneumoniae* isolated were penicillin nonsusceptible (minimal inhibitory concentration [MIC] > 0.10 μg/mL). This increasing resistance might alter the efficacy of some of the frequently used topical antibiotics. There thus continues to be debate on the optimal use of topical agents in the treatment of bacterial conjunctivitis. Many ophthalmologists now avoid the aminoglycoside or sulfa-containing agents, reporting that they often hurt when applied and frequently have lower efficacy against the increasingly resistant pathogens. These specialists often recommend proceeding directly to a topical fluoroquinolone if treatment is to be offered.

Otitis-Conjunctivitis Syndrome

In the early 1980s, it was recognized that there was a unique pediatric syndrome of conjunctivitis and otitis media.

Etiology

The pathogen in this clinical syndrome is thought to be nontypeable *H. influenzae*.

Presentation

Children usually present after development of conjunctivitis with low-grade fever and mild respiratory symptoms. Several days later, otitis media becomes apparent, usually with the development of ear pain.

Diagnosis

Diagnosis is made by the typical history and documentation of otitis media closely following an episode of conjunctivitis.

Management

The treatment of the otitis-conjunctivitis syndrome has also been the subject of considerable investigation. About 25% of children who present with *H. influenzae* conjunctivitis who are treated topically ultimately develop otitis media. In one study, the administration of ampicillin to patients presenting initially with purulent conjunctivitis alone resulted in fewer episodes of secondary otitis media. Interestingly, a subsequent study using cefixime did not show a similar benefit in preventing otitis media. Patients who present with both otitis and conjunctivitis at initial evaluation deserve systemic therapy, typically an oral antibiotic that covers β-lactamase–producing *H. influenzae*. Some recommend that oral antibiotics be used in children who present with bacterial conjunctivitis and who are considered at high risk for otitis media (i.e., young age, attendance at daycare). If systemic therapy is given, topical therapy is not needed.

Periorbital Cellulitis

Epidemiology and Etiology

Direct inoculation of pathogens into the skin and soft tissue around the eye are common. Bacterial pathogens may be introduced secondary to insect bite or mild trauma with resultant periorbital cellulitis. Organisms most frequently causing these infections are *Streptococcus pyogenes* and *Staphylococcus aureus*.

Presentation

Affected children present with periorbital cellulitis and swelling. Frequently, there is a readily observed cut or break in the skin accompanied by impetiginous lesions about the face. Extraocular movements are typically normal.

Diagnosis

Diagnosis is based on the physical examination. A culture of an accompanying discharge from a cut or area of trauma may yield the responsible pathogen.

Management

If this mechanism is suspected, antibiotic therapy should be geared to these particular organisms. Clindamycin or a first-generation cephalosporin offers good coverage.

MECHANISM OF HEMATOGENOUS SPREAD

Epidemiology and Etiology

> Periorbital cellulitis can also occur when periorbital regions become seeded during bacteremia.

The classic bacteria associated with bacteremic periorbital cellulitis are *H. influenzae*, (type b) and *S. pneumoniae*. It is thought that there is a predilection for these bacteremic organisms to deposit within the periorbital area; it is also possible that sinusitis with either of these organisms can infect periorbital regions as a result of venous congestion and decreased lymphatic flow.

Presentation

Bacteremic patients often present in the first 5 years of life. They have periorbital cellulitis and swelling, although there is no obvious cut or area of inoculation.

Diagnosis

Yield of blood cultures in bacteremic periorbital cellulitis is about 25%. The diagnosis is often suspected in a child with periorbital cellulitis and no obvious signs or history of preceding trauma.

Management

In a child younger than 5 years of age with periorbital cellulitis in whom there is no obvious trauma, antibiotic coverage should include those agents active against either *H. influenzae* or *S. pneumoniae*. Second- or third-generation cephalosporins are adequate for this purpose. The conjugate vaccine for *H. influenzae* has led to a great decrease in the incidence of *Haemophilus* disease; it is also possible that the introduction of the Prevnar vaccine will cause a similar decrease in pneumococcal bacteremia and subsequent pneumococcal periorbital cellulitis.

A common question arises regarding the need for lumbar puncture in patients with presumed hematogenous periorbital cellulitis. These patients may be at risk for meningitis because the bacteremia that has localized in the periorbital regions may also have seeded in the cerebrospinal fluid. The rate of concurrent meningitis seen with *H. influenzae* periorbital cellulitis is about 5%. Lumbar puncture is recommended in younger children, especially those younger than 12 months of age and those with associated irritability or meningeal findings. Any abnormal findings on cerebrospinal fluid, such as a pleocytosis with neutrophil predominance, warrants treatment of presumed meningitis.

MECHANISM OF CONTIGUOUS SPREAD (ORBITAL CELLULITIS)

Epidemiology and Etiology

The ethmoid sinuses form the medial walls of the orbit. Children with significant ethmoid sinusitis may have spread of infection into the orbit. The organisms involved in such cases are the organisms of sinusitis; *S. aureus*, group A streptococcus, *S. pneumoniae*, *H. influenzae*, and anaerobic bacteria.

Presentation

Typically, the patient with orbital cellulitis is older. There is no evidence of direct inoculation. Parents often give a history of a preceding sinus infection. There is often proptosis and limitation of the extraocular movements.

It is important to realize that periorbital cellulitis is caused by a different mechanism than orbital cellulitis and thus will not progress to orbital cellulitis. A comparison of the features of periorbital and orbital cellulitis can be found in Table 8.1.

In a child with a red swollen eye and an exam consistent with contiguous spread from a sinus infection, evaluation for extension into the orbit is essential. It is important to remember that purulent infection can spread into the orbit and affect orbital structures, particularly the optic nerve.

Diagnosis

Examination should determine whether there is proptosis or a decrease in extraocular movements. Visual acuity should, if possible, be tested. It is understood that in patients with this condition, the eye can be swollen to such an extent that examination can be difficult. In this case, the radiographic procedure of choice is computed tomography (CT) of the orbit. This exam will show clearly the orbital structures and the presence of orbital disease (Fig. 8.1).

Management

A useful staging system has been published for orbital cellulitis (Chandler's criteria). As in many staging criteria, the identification of a particular stage has been correlated with the need for particular management.

TABLE 8.1. *Periorbital Versus Orbital Cellulitis*

1. Periorbital cellulitis	a. <5 years
	b. Mechanism
	1. Trauma
	2. Bacteremia
	c. Ocular motility not affected
	d. Organisms
	1. Trauma *Streptococcus pyogenes*
	Staphylococcus aureus
	2. Bacteremia *Streptococcus pneumoniae*
	e. Progression to orbital disease does *not* occur
2. Orbital cellulitis	a. >12 years
	b. Mechanism—sinusitis
	c. Ocular motility may be reduced
	d. Organism *S. pneumoniae*
	Nontypeable *Haemophilus* species
	Moraxella catarrhalis
	S. aureus
	e. Treatment may include surgical drainage

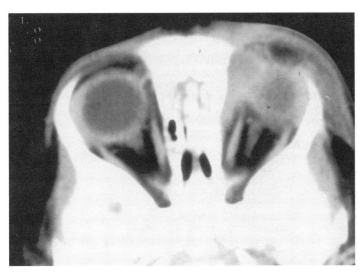

FIG. 8.1. Computed tomography scan of orbit showing left orbital abscess.

Chandler's Stages of Orbital Cellulitis

Stage 1: Periorbital cellulitis. Eyelid swelling with sinusitis. No intraocular disease.

Stage 2: Edema of the orbital lining with proptosis and limitation of extraocular movement. No subperiosteal abscess seen within orbit.

Stage 3: Visual loss, progression of changes seen in stage 2, with subperiosteal abscess and globe displacement within orbit.

Stage 4: Ophthalmoplegia with visual loss. CT scan shows proptosis and abscess formation involving the extraocular muscles and orbital fat.

Traditionally, Chandler's stage 4 orbital cellulitis had been considered a surgical condition. Recently, case studies have been collected that suggest that even patients with well-defined subperiosteal abscesses may respond to intravenous antibiotics without the need for surgical drainage. Antibiotics to cover all possible organisms would include nafcillin and a third-generation cephalosporin. Clindamycin can be substituted for nafcillin because it is effective against *S. pneumoniae* and *S. aureus* and also provides coverage for anaerobic bacteria. Another possible choice is ampicillin-sulbactam (Unasyn). Most specialists believe that patients with significant intraorbital abscesses need close monitoring. Serial examination, including assessment of vision, extraocular muscle function, and re-

TABLE 8.2. *Management of the Swollen Eye*

1. Conjunctivitis
   a. Ophthalmia neonatorium
      i) Pathogens: *Neisseria gonorrhoeae*
                    Chlamydia trachomatis
      ii) Treatment: Ceftriaxone, 50–75 mg/kg/d in 1 or 2 divided doses. Oral erythromycin needed (50 mg/kg/d in 4 divided doses) if *C. trachomatis* is present
   b. Bacterial conjunctivitis (toddlers)
      i) Pathogens: Nontypeable *Haemophilus influenzae*
                    Streptococcus pneumoniae
                    Adenovirus
      ii) Topical treatment: Polytrim (trimethoprim sulfate and polymyxin)
                             Gentamycin sulfate
                             Sodium sulfacetamide
                             Ciprofloxacin (Ciloxan)
   c. Otitis–conjunctivitis syndrome
      i) Pathogen: Nontypeable *H. influenzae*
      ii) Treatment: Amoxicillin-clavulanate (Augmentin)
                     Oral second- or third-generation cephalosporins
2. Periorbital cellulitis (bacteremic spread)
   a. Pathogens: *H. influenzae*, type b
      S. pneumoniae
   b. Treatment: second- or third-generation cephalosporins
3. Orbital cellulitis (contagious spread)
   a. Pathogens: *H. influenzae, S. pneumonia, Staphylococcus aureus*, anaerobes
   b. Medical treatment
      i) Unasyn (ampicillin-sulbactam), 100–200 mg/kg/day of ampicillin component
      ii) Clindamycin, 40 mg/kg/d in three divided doses in combination with third-generation cephalosporin
   c. Surgical drainage should be strongly considered

peat CT, are mandatory. Failure to improve within 24 to 48 hours remains an indication for surgical drainage. Because the mechanism of infection includes extension through the ethmoid sinus, many infectious disease specialists recommend treating orbital cellulitis as an osteomyelitis. A minimum of 21 days of therapy is recommended (Table 8.2).

SELECTED READINGS

Block SL, Hedrick J, Tyler R, et al. Increasing bacterial resistance in pediatric acute conjunctivitis (1997–1998). *Antimicrob Agents Chemother* 2000;44(6):1650–1654.
Givner LB. Periorbital versus orbital cellulitis. *Pediatr Infect Dis J* 2002;21(12):1157–1158.
Harrison CJ, Hedrick JA, Block SL. Relation of the outcome of the conjunctivitis-otitis syndrome to identifiable risk factors and oral antimicrobial therapy. *Pediatr Infect Dis J* 1987;(6):536–540.
Ruttum MS, Ogawa G. Adenoviral conjunctivitis mimics preseptal and orbital cellulitis in young children. *Pediatr Infect Dis J* 1996;15(3):266–267.
Starkey CR, Steele RW. Medical management of orbital cellulitis. *Pediatr Infect Dis J* 2001;20(10)1002–1005.
Teoh DL, Reynolds S. Diagnosis and management of pediatric conjunctivitis. *Pediatr Emerg Care* 2003;19(1):48–55.
Wald ER. Conjunctivitis in infants and children. *Pediatr Infect Dis J* 1997;16:[2 Suppl]S17–20.

9

Cervical Adenitis

Swelling of cervical lymph nodes is a common pediatric problem.

The differential diagnosis of cervical adenitis is extensive and includes acute and chronic infections, Kawasaki syndrome, and malignancy. The evaluation process should be logical with the history and physical guiding the subsequent workup.

ACUTE INFECTIONS ASSOCIATED WITH CERVICAL ADENITIS

Etiology (Bacterial)

The most common bacterial cause of acute unilateral cervical adenopathy is infection with *Staphylococcus aureus* or *Streptococcus pyogenes* (group A streptococci). These two organisms are the cause of acute unilateral disease in more than 80% of cases.

Presentation

There is often sudden onset of fever, swelling, tenderness, and overlying erythema.

Diagnosis

Diagnosis of acute bacterial adenitis is typically made by the clinical history and examination.

Management

Therapy is with an antibiotic with activity against both *S. aureus* and group A streptococci. A first generation cephalosporin or clindamycin can be used. Children who appear toxic with high fever and decreased oral intake may need to be managed initially as inpatients; for these children, ampicillin-sulbactam (Unasyn) is a good intravenous agent. It is often difficult to predict in a particular patient which nodes will suppurate and thus require surgical drainage. Serial exams and the use of computed tomography of the neck are helpful in determining whether the child will require surgery (Fig. 9.1). Once the child is afebrile and taking fluids well, these serial examinations can be done as an outpatient while on oral antibiotics.

The traditional surgical approach to suppurative cervical adenitis that had failed to respond completely to medical management was open incision and drainage. Drawbacks to this technique included the need for general anesthesia and a large scar. There is increasing experience with needle aspiration in the surgical management of suppurative cervical adenitis. The advantage of needle aspiration over incisional drainage is that general anesthesia may not be required and surgical scarring may be minimized. Many pediatric surgeons are now using this technique as a first-line method for suppurative adenitis unresponsive to antibiotic treatment (Table 9.1).

Etiology (Viral)

Acute bilateral cervical lymphadenitis is frequently caused by viral infections, including Epstein-Barr virus, cytomegalovirus, and adenovirus.

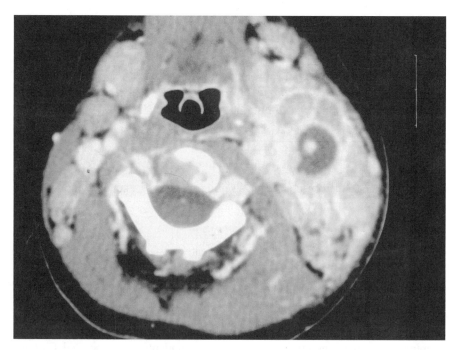

FIG. 9.1. Computed tomograph revealing cervical adenitis with abscess formation (see color plate).

TABLE 9.1. *Causes of Acute Bacterial Cervical Adenitis*

Acute infection (*Staphylococcus aureus, Streptococcus pyogenes*)
1. Associated with fever, erythema, tenderness
2. May proceed to suppuration and require incisional drainage
3. Outpatient therapy
   Cephalexin (Keflex), 25–50 mg/kg/d in 4 divided doses
   Clindamycin, 20–40 mg/kg/d in 3 divided doses
   Augmentin (amoxicillin-clavulanate), 25–45 mg/kg/d; for children <40 kg
4. Inpatient therapy
   Ampicillin-sulbactam (Unasyn), 100–200 mg/kg/d of ampicillin component divided q6h

Presentation

Patients often have associated cough and rhinorrhea.

Diagnosis

Diagnosis of viral adenopathy is usually made clinically, based on associated symptoms and the absence of fever and erythema, which characterize acute bacterial disease.

Management

Care in these cases is supportive. It is important to realize that after a viral infection, the lymph node enlargement may persist for many weeks, even though the acute symptoms of fever, cough, and coryza have resolved.

CHRONIC INFECTIONS ASSOCIATED WITH CERVICAL ADENITIS

The two major causes of chronic infectious lymphadenitis in children are nontuberculous mycobacteria and cat-scratch disease. Additional causes of chronic infectious lymphadenopathy include toxoplasmosis and actinomycosis.

Nontuberculous Mycobacteria

Etiology

Nontuberculous mycobacteria (NTM) is a common cause of chronic cervical lymphadenitis in children. The nontuberculous mycobacterium that most often causes pediatric adenopathy is *Mycobacterium avium-intracellulare* (MAI). These organisms are ubiquitous in nature, often found in soil and contaminated water. The mycobacteria enter the oral cavity and may infect cervical lymph nodes. Although disseminated MAI is a common illness in end-stage acquired immunodeficiency disease (AIDS) patients, adenopathy in pediatrics is not considered a symptom of underlying immunodeficiency.

Presentation

Patients present with chronic lymph node enlargement over several weeks to months, although occasionally acute infection is seen. Affected nodes progress to fluctuation with an accompanying overlying violaceous color (Fig. 9.2). Without treatment, these nodes often rupture and develop sinus tracts.

Diagnosis

NTM infection should be considered in any patient with progressive adenitis not responding to traditional antibiotics. Needle aspiration often shows white blood cells but with negative Gram stain and culture. Tuberculin skin testing for *Mycobacterium tuberculosis* (MTB) may reveal a small degree of induration because MTB shares certain antigens with MAI. There is currently no skin test approved by the U.S. Food and Drug Administration (FDA) specifically for NTM. Children with MAI adenitis have negative chest x-rays and are **not** contagious.

Management

NTM are not susceptible to traditional antituberculous medications. For this reason, the treatment of MAI adenitis is complete surgical excision of the affected

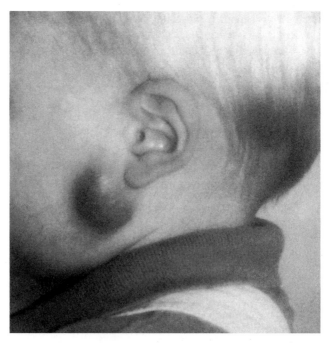

FIG. 9.2. Chronic cervical adenitis seen in atypical mycobacterial infection. (see color plate).

node. Excisional biopsy is both diagnostic and therapeutic. The use of fine-needle aspiration or incision and drainage should be avoided because they can help facilitate formation of chronic fistula. The gold standard for the diagnosis of NTM adenitis is culture of the organism. Because growth of acid-fast bacteria may take several weeks, there has been some investigation regarding whether the histopathology of the excised node can help differentiate infections caused by NTM from MTB. Features associated with NTM infection include lack of significant caseation and less defined granuloma formation. There are instances in which the clinician will need to start antituberculous therapy pending final culture results.

In the cases in which complete excision is not possible because of extensive disease, medical therapy can be attempted. For *Mycobacterium avium* complex, a macrolide antibiotic such as clarithromycin or azithromycin, combined with ethambutol, is recommended.

Mycobacterium tuberculosis

Etiology

MTB is an unusual cause of cervical adenitis in developed countries. Transmission is person to person, with initial infection caused by aerosolized bacteria. After deposition in pulmonary alveoli, mycobacteria can travel through the lymphatic vessels to cervical lymph nodes.

Presentation of MTB adenitis can be similar to adenitis from NTM, with chronic infection progressing to purplish discoloration and fistula formation.

Diagnosis

Major distinguishing points of NTB adenitis include purified protein derivative (PPD), which often has greater than 15 mm of induration. Chest radiographs may reveal hilar adenopathy. Excisional biopsy and culture are often needed for definitive diagnosis.

Management

Unlike NTM adenitis, treatment is medical with at least two antituberculous medications effective against the mycobacteria (see chapter 12).

Cat-Scratch Disease

Etiology

Another common cause of chronic adenopathy in children is cat-scratch disease. This infection is caused by *Bartonella henselae*. The organisms are introduced through the skin by a cat scratch or bite; the most commonly affected area is the upper extremity, resulting in epitrochlear or axillary node enlargement.

Presentation

Lymphadenopathy is the most common presentation of cat-scratch disease. A scratch to the facial area may cause significant cervical lymphadenopathy. *B. henselae* can also cause additional clinical syndromes, including aseptic meningitis and encephalitis. Parinaud oculoglandular syndrome is infection with *B. henselae* following inoculation of the conjunctiva and presents with conjunctivitis and periauricular adenopathy.

Diagnosis

A history of cat exposure should always be elicited in evaluation of chronic cervical adenitis. Diagnosis can be confirmed by serology using indirect immunofluorescence antibody (IFA). Immunoglobulin G (IgG) antibody titers higher than 1:512 have been reported to suggest acute infection. IgM antibodies against *B. henselae* have been found only infrequently in the early stages of cat-scratch disease. Polymerase chain reaction analysis of a lymph node aspirate or biopsy can be performed, although *B. henselae* DNA may be present in lymph nodes only in the first weeks of illness.

Management

Most patients with cat-scratch disease have spontaneous resolution. There is no consensus on the use of antibiotics for cat-scratch disease. There have been reports that oral antibiotics, including macrolides, trimethoprim-sulfamethoxazole, and ciprofloxacin, may be effective. A single randomized and double-blind placebo-controlled study found that a 5-day course of oral azithromycin resulted in significant reduction in lymphadenopathy caused by cat-scratch disease when patients were treated within the first month of illness. Needle aspiration can be used for nodes that are suppurative and painful. Unlike chronic adenitis from NTM, surgical excision is generally neither needed nor advised.

Toxoplasma gondii

Etiology

T. gondii is an intracellular protozoan that is acquired by contact with cats or consumption of undercooked meats. Toxoplasmosis eventually infects a significant portion of the adult population.

Presentation

Patients who become symptomatic with this infection often have fever, sore throat, and posterior cervical adenopathy. Nodes may be mildly tender but as a rule do not progress to fluctuance. Toxoplasmosis adenopathy can persist for several months. The clinical course is usually benign and self-limited in the immunocompetent host.

Diagnosis

Toxoplasmosis adenitis can be diagnosed serologically. Biopsy of affected nodes reveals characteristic features, including epithelioid cells that encroach on the margins of lymphoid germinal centers.

Management

No treatment is usually required in patients with normal immune function.

Actinomycosis

Etiology

Actinomyces species are gram-positive bacilli that are acid-fast negative. They are part of the gastrointestinal tract flora and can cause infection following oral or facial trauma.

Presentation

Actinomyces species causes three major categories of disease, including cervicofacial, thoracic, and abdominal. Cervicofacial disease is the most common manifestation and often occurs after facial trauma or dental procedures. The typical presentation is progressive swelling and development of a "woody," lumpy jaw not responsive to traditional antibiotics. There is increasing appreciation that cervical facial actinomycosis may often be a polymicrobial process. *S. aureus* or group A streptococci may be involved as a co-pathogen in the development of cervicofacial disease; when this occurs, an acute painful abscess or cellulitis may be the initial manifestation. Actinomycosis should be considered in the proper setting, particularly with progressive cervical adenopathy present in a patient following significant dental work or facial trauma.

Diagnosis

Biopsy of the affected area reveals beaded and branched acid-fast negative grampositive bacilli. Sulfur granules are present in about 25% of cases and can be visualized in biopsy specimens. Culture of actinomycosis is difficult, and often the Gram stain and biopsy findings suggest the correct diagnosis.

Management

Therapy of actinomycosis involves high-dose intravenous penicillin G, 100,000 to 250,000 units/kg per day in four divided doses for several months, followed by oral penicillin, clindamycin, or tetracycline. Duration of therapy is 6 to 12 months. Surgical drainage may be needed for cases that do not respond to appropriate antimicrobials.

Major Chronic Infections of Cervical Adenitis

1. Nontuberculous mycobacteria (MAI)
   a. Associated with purplish discoloration, sinus tract formation
   b. PPD < 10 mm induration
   c. Excisional biopsy
2. Cat-scratch disease
   a. Caused by *Bartonella henselae*
   b. Diagnosis
      i. Serology
      ii. Biopsy reveals stellate abscesses
   c. Treatment: azithromycin
   d. Needle aspiration
3. Mycobacterium tuberculosis
   a. Rare in developed countries
   b. PPD > 15 mm induration
   c. Positive chest x-ray
   d. Medical therapy

NONINFECTIOUS CAUSES OF CERVICAL ADENOPATHY

Kawasaki syndrome

Etiology

Kawasaki syndrome is an acute inflammatory illness of unknown etiology. The original term for Kawasaki syndrome was the *mucocutaneous lymph node syndrome*, and cervical adenitis can be a feature of this illness. Most children diagnosed with Kawasaki syndrome are younger than 5 years of age.

Presentation

The cause of Kawasaki syndrome is unknown; therefore, the diagnosis is based on clinical criteria. The diagnostic criteria include fever, edema and erythema of the palms and soles, nonpurulent conjunctivitis, redness of the lips, strawberry tongue, cervical adenitis, and a skin rash. It is not uncommon for patients with Kawasaki syndrome to present initially with a unilateral cervical adenitis, only to progress to the full manifestation of the syndrome. It is for this reason that children with unilateral cervical adenitis who have continued fever despite appropriate antibiotics should be evaluated with the Kawasaki syndrome criteria in mind.

Diagnosis

Diagnosis of Kawasaki syndrome is made by having five of the six clinical criteria and by exclusion of other syndromes such as viral illnesses or toxin-producing bacterial disease. Additional non-criteria signs of Kawasaki disease, including sterile pyuria, marked elevation of the sedimentation rate, and early growing desquamation, are frequently helpful in the diagnosis. Thrombocytosis and palmar desquamation after the first 2 weeks of illness are also characteristic.

A recent study suggested that the cervical lymph nodes in Kawasaki disease may have specific ultrasonographic features; ultrasound appearance of the inflamed nodes in Kawasaki syndrome is often a mass of multiple hypoechoic nodes resembling a cluster of grapes. This is distinct from the ultrasound features of routine bacterial lymphadenitis and can be helpful in patient evaluation.

The management of Kawasaki syndrome includes the use of intravenous immune globulin (IVIG) at a dose of 2 mg/kg. High-dose aspirin, 80 to 100 mg/kg per day in four divided doses, is used until the patient has resolution of fever. The patient is then maintained on low-dose aspirin, 3 to 5 mg/kg per day for about 6 weeks until platelet count and sedimentation rate become normal.

Malignant Causes of Cervical Adenopathy

Etiology

The possibility of malignancy in a child with enlarged nodes is always present in the minds of caretakers. There has been considerable effort made to define those children whose enlarged lymph nodes may be caused by a malignancy such as Hodgkin's disease, non-Hodgkin's lymphoma, or leukemia.

Presentation

Up to 30% of children whose adenopathy is caused by a malignancy have associated fever, anorexia, and weight loss. Additional factors associated with malignancy include an abnormal chest x-ray and increasing node size. Eosinophilia can also be seen in patients with Hodgkin's disease. Extreme elevation of sedimentation rate, uric acid, and lactate dehydrogenase (LDH) can be seen. A frequently quoted study from the early 1980s found that children with supraclavicular adenopathy, unexplained weight loss, or fixation of the lymph node to overlying

Table 9.2. *Noninfectious Causes of Cervical Adenitis*

Cause	Comments

1. Kawasaki disease	1. Criteria include 5/6 of the following:
	  a. Fever greater than 5 days
	  b. Nonpurulent conjunctivitis
	  c. Swollen palms, feet
	  d. Cervical arthritis
	  e. Rash
	  f. Erythematous mucous membranes

2. Malignancy	1. Associated with
	  a. Unexplained fever
	  b. Unexplained weight loss
	  c. Fixation of node to overlying skin
	  d. Supraclavicular adenopathy
	  e. Eosinophilia

skin have a high likelihood of malignant disease and should be considered for early biopsy.

Diagnosis

The diagnosis of malignancy always requires biopsy.

Management

Therapy is dependent on the particular malignancy diagnosed (Table 9.2).

EVALUATION OF PEDIATRIC LYMPHADENOPATHY

Testing starts with a complete history and physical examination. Duration of the lymphadenopathy, along with associated symptoms, including fever, anorexia, weight loss, and animal exposure, should always be obtained. Examination of the child should be focused on the enlarged lymph node, whether it is red, tender, or fluctuant and associated organomegaly and lymphadenopathy at other areas.

If a node is consistent with an acute bacterial infection, oral antibiotics can be given. If the clinical picture suggests a more chronic condition, laboratory evaluation can include a complete blood count with differential and a metabolic panel including LDH and uric acid. Chest x-ray looking for hilar adenopathy, along with a tuberculous skin testing, is also helpful. Serology for particular pathogens, including toxoplasmosis and cat-scratch disease, may be obtained as suggested by the history.

Ultimately, nodes that remain enlarged and whose etiology is not defined need to be considered for excisional biopsy. Fine-needle aspiration is frequently used to evaluate adenopathy in the adult population. Pediatric specialists are less enthusiastic about this procedure because a significant number of fine-needle aspirations in children do not obtain tissue for appropriate pathology and diagnostic studies (Table 9.3).

Table 9.3. *Evaluation of Pediatric Cervical Adenitis*

1. History
   Duration of lymph node swelling
   Associated symptoms/ fever, weight loss, pallor, bruising
   Travel history (Endemic areas for tuberculosis)
   Exposure history (cats)
2. Examinations
   Associated nodes (particularly supraclavicular)
   Organomegaly
   Tenderness; erythema of node
   Associated criteria for Kawasaki disease
3. Evaluation
   Chest x-ray
   Complete blood count, sedimentation rate, metabolic panel
   Purified protein derivative
   Serologies (as suggested by history)
      Epstein-Barr virus
      Cytomegalovirus
      Cat-scratch disease
      Toxoplasmosis
Biopsy

SELECTED READINGS

Knight PJ, Mulne AF, Vaggy LE. When is lymph node biopsy indicated in children with enlarged peripheral nodes? *Pediatrics* 1982;69(4):391–396.

Peters TR, Edward KM. Cervical lymphadenopathy and adenitis. *Pediatr Rev* 2000;21(12)399–405.

Ridder GJ, Boedeker CC, Technau-Ihling K, et al. Role of cat-scratch disease in lymphadenopathy in the head and neck. *Clin Infect Dis* 2002;35(6):643–649.

Serour F, Gorenstein A, Somekh E. Needle aspiration for suppurative cervical adenitis. *Clin Pediatr* 2002;41(7):471–4744.

Tashiro N, Matsubara T, Uchida M, et al Ultrasonographic evaluation of cervical lymph nodes in Kawasaki disease. *Pediatrics* 2002;09(5):E77.

Twist CJ, Link MP. Assessment of lymphadenopathy in children. *Pediatr Clin North Am* 2002;49(5): 1009–1025.

10

Urinary Tract Infections

The diagnosis of pediatric urinary tract infection is important because pediatric urinary tract infection can be a manifestation of underlying urinary tract abnormalities. Failure to recognize and appropriately manage these abnormalities may lead to recurrent urinary tract infection, renal scarring, and long-term alterations in renal function.

ETIOLOGY

Pediatric urinary tract infection begins with colonization of the periurethral area with gastrointestinal bacteria. These bacteria may then ascend into the bladder, kidneys, or both. A variety of virulence factors may promote infection with certain bacterial isolates. *Escherichia coli* organisms, a primary cause of urinary tract infection, have a variety of adhesive molecules that facilitate binding to uroepithelial cells. These "pili" function as ladders that enable the bacteria to ascend from the periurethral area into the urinary tract.

Host factors may also play a role in the development of complicated urinary tract infection. Ascension of bacteria from the bladder into the renal parenchyma may be facilitated by vesicoureteral reflux (VUR). VUR is a congenital condition resulting from a defect in the ureterovesical junction. This defect affects closure of the ureter, which then allows retrograde flow of urine from the bladder into the kidneys. Infection with *E. coli* accounts for most urinary tract infections. Less common pathogens include enterococcus and other enterics such as *Proteus* species.

PRESENTATION

In adults, the diagnosis of urinary tract infection is often associated with signs such as increased frequency or dysuria; these symptoms may be lacking in young children. A urinary tract infection needs to be considered in any young child presenting with fever. Studies have shown that the rate of urinary tract infection in infants with unexplained fever is between 5% and 10%. An uncircumcised male with an unexplained fever of greater than 39°C (102.2°F) has been reported as having a 35% chance of having a urinary tract infection.

DIAGNOSIS

Paramount to the diagnosis of urinary tract infection and any subsequent radiographic investigation is proper collection and examination of the urine. A bagged specimen is not appropriate for the diagnosis of urinary tract infection because it is easily contaminated by bacteria. In infants who are in diapers, an "in-and-out" catheterization is usually required. In toilet-trained children, a clean-catch specimen may be adequate if the child can be adequately prepped. Urine specimens that cannot be processed at once should be refrigerated at 4°C. Urine kept at room temperature, for even a short period of time, can alter the results of leukocyte esterase and nitrate tests routinely done on dipstick examination.

Analysis of a properly obtained urine specimen can provide a clue to the presence of infection. However, there remains considerable debate about the best test to perform. Urine dipstick for nitrate and leukocyte esterase, evaluation for bacteriuria, and the presence of pyuria have all been used as screening tests for urinary tract infections.

Nitrate detected by dipstick is positive in 50% of children with urinary tract infection. This relatively low figure may be related to the fact that the test requires bacteria to remain in the bladder for several hours, a condition that is less likely in children.

The evaluation for pyuria is complicated by a variety of factors, including the precise number of white blood cells needed for presumptive diagnosis of infection and whether the urine specimen being evaluated is centrifuged before analysis. Hemocytometry is a method used to count white blood cells in body fluids such as spinal fluid and urine. In recent years, considerable study has been done on the use of hemocytometry in "enhanced urinalysis." In this method, urine is obtained by catheter and evaluated as an uncentrifuged specimen. The enhanced urinalysis is considered positive if there are more than 10 white blood cells/mm^3 and any bacteria on Gram stain. The sensitivity of this method is 85%, with a specificity of 99%. The drawback to enhanced urinalysis is that the equipment needed may not be readily available. The traditional standard urinalysis uses centrifuged specimens, with pyuria being defined as at least 5 white blood cells per high-power field and the presence of any bacteria. The sensitivity of this method is 65%, with 92% specificity.

In 1999, the American Academy of Pediatrics recommended dipstick evaluation, standard microscopy, and Gram stain as useful screens for urinary tract infection. Positive leukocyte esterase or nitrate on dipstick, greater than 5 white blood cells per high-power field on standard urinalysis, or a positive Gram stain of unspun urine is suggestive of urinary tract infection. These parameters continue to be evaluated, with some investigators commenting on the need to evaluate further the screening methods or even to eliminate urinalysis entirely. It should be understood that urine testing serves as a screen. A negative screen does not rule out urinary tract infection. Clinical correlation is always needed. In a febrile child who has a strong possibility of urinary tract infection, a negative urinalysis should be followed by a urine culture.

Use of Urine Culture

A urine culture is obtained by inoculating a culture media with a standard volume of urine, typically 0.01 mL. Colony forming units (CFUs) are then calculated by counting the number of colonies on the inoculated area and converting it to CFU/mL. Most children who have urinary tract infections have bacterial colony counts of more than 10^5 CFU/mL of urine. This cutoff valve was established through studies in adults, with few comparable studies having been performed in children. There have been published guidelines to redefine the criteria for pediatric patients correlated with a variety of techniques for urine collection. Bacterial colony counts of more than 10^5 CFU/mL of urine collected by the clean-catch method correlated with high likelihood of a urinary tract infection. For catheter-obtained specimens, 5×10^4 CFU/mL is considered significant. In children who have had urine obtained by suprapubic aspiration, most investigators believe that the presence of any gram-negative enteric organism qualifies as a urinary tract infection.

Diagnosis of Urinary Tract Infection

Collection	Likely urinary tract infection
a. Suprapubic	Any gram-negative organism
b. Clean voided	
Boy	$>10^5$ CFU/mL of urine
Girl	$>10^5$ CFU/mL of urine
c. Catheter obtained	5×10^4 CFU/mL of urine

MANAGEMENT OF URINARY TRACT INFECTION

In children who are not toxic and can maintain hydration, oral antibiotics can be started. Traditional oral antibiotics for the treatment of urinary tract infection in children include amoxicillin, trimethoprim-sulfamethoxazole, and oral cephalosporins. The increasing resistance of *E. coli* to amoxicillin has reduced empiric therapy with this antibiotic. The newer-generation oral cephalosporins, such as cefixime, cefdinir, and ceftibuten, have excellent gram-negative enteric bacteria coverage and can be useful in the treatment of resistant *E. coli* urinary tract infections. Nitrofurantoin has been used for the treatment of cystitis, although its failure to achieve good bloodstream concentrations has led to the recommendation that it should not be used to treat febrile infants or children with upper urinary tract involvement. The total duration of therapy for a urinary tract infection is variable, although patients typically receive 7 to 14 days of therapy.

RADIOGRAPHIC EVALUATION AFTER URINARY TRACT INFECTION

Imaging of the infant and young child with a urinary tract infection is one of the fundamentals of pediatrics. Urinary tract infection in children can be a manifestation of underlying urinary tract abnormalities that need to be documented. The American Academy of Pediatrics recommends that imaging of the urinary tract be done for every child 2 months to 2 years of age after the first urinary tract infection, regardless of the sex of the child.

Renal Ultrasound

The use of ultrasound can document hydronephrosis and ureteral dilation secondary to obstruction. The American Academy of Pediatrics has recommended the use of renal ultrasonogram for young children after the first urinary tract infection. This test should be done promptly in young children, particularly those who do not respond quickly to antimicrobial therapy. Young boys are at particular risk for posterior ureteral valves, and ultrasonography can be used to document quickly this malformation and the presence of accompanying hydronephrosis. Recently, the use of ultrasonography has been questioned by a variety of investigators. In a recent study of more than 300 children with urinary tract infection, ultrasound results were normal in almost 90% of cases; those that were abnormal did not modify patient management.

Cystourethrography

Voiding cystourethrography (VCUG) is still considered a useful test. The VCUG is performed by placing a catheter through the urethra into the bladder and instilling an iodinated contrast. Although this test is uncomfortable for the patient, it is the only method for diagnosing VUR. VUR is graded according to an international grading system. Scores increase with increasing ureteral dilation and progressive filling of the upper urinary tracts. VUR is identified in up to 50% of children who are evaluated after the first documented urinary tract infection.

The traditional recommendation was to obtain the VCUG about 4 weeks after the diagnosis of urinary tract infection. The logic for this recommendation was that acute infection and the acute inflammatory state of the upper urinary tract system would lead to a transient reflux. The current thinking regarding VUR is that it is a primary congenital phenomenon and not related to infection. For this reason, many clinicians obtain the VCUG on a more urgent basis after documentation of urine sterilization.

TABLE 10.1. *Pediatric Urinary Tract Infection*

Treatment
  1. Parental
Cefotaxime (Claforan), 100–200 mg/kg/d divided q8h
    Ceftriaxone (Rocephin), 50–75 mg/kg/d divided q12
    Ampicillin (if enterococcus is a possibility), 100–200 mg/kg/d in 4 divided doses
  2. Oral
    Amoxicillin, 40mg/kg/d in 3 divided doses
    Trimethoprim-sulfamethoxazole (Bactrim), 8–10mg/kg/d of trimethoprim component
      divided q12h
    Cephalexin (Keflex), 25–50 mg/kg/d in 4 divided doses
    Cefpodoxime (Vantin), 10mg/kg/d divided q12–24h
Imaging
  1. Renal ultrasound
  2. Voiding cystourethrogram
  3. DMSA scanning
Prophylaxis
  1. Nitrofurantoin (Furadantin), 1–2 mg/kg/dose PO qhs; maximum dose, 100 mg
  2. Trimethoprim-sulfamethoxazole (Bactrim), 2–4 mg/kg/day PO qd

DMSA, dimercaptosuccinic acid.

Renal Scintigraphy

Another study available to pediatricians for the evaluation of urinary tract infection is renal scintigraphy. Dimercaptosuccinic acid (DMSA) is attached to technetium and then infused into a patient. This compound localizes in renal tubules and can be used to diagnose acute pyelonephritis (sensitivity about 90%). DMSA scan can also be used to assess renal scarring months after acute infection. This test is useful if the diagnosis of pyelonephritis is in doubt or as a tool to follow patients with high-grade VUR and chronic infections.

MANAGEMENT OF VESICOURETERAL REFLUX

Most infants with documented vesicoureteral reflux ultimately outgrow this condition. Reflux of sterile urine is not thought to cause renal damage; thus, antibiotic prophylaxis is given to prevent recurrent infection and the continuing reflux of infected urine, which may cause renal scarring. Prophylaxis with either trimethoprim-sulfamethoxazole or nitrofurantoin is frequently used. It should be remembered that breakthrough infections are always possible because of either noncompliance or the acquisition of resistant organisms not covered by the antibiotics being used for prophylaxis. A febrile illness in a child receiving prophylaxis for a urinary tract infection always warrants urinalysis and urine culture as part of the evaluation.

A summary of the diagnosis, treatment, and subsequent imaging can be seen in Table 10.1.

SELECTED READINGS

American Academy of Pediatrics. Committee of Quality Improvement. Subcommittee of Urinary Tract Infection. Practice parameter on the diagnosis, treatment, and evaluation of the initial urinary tract infection in febrile infants and young children. *Pediatrics* 1999;103(4 Pt. 1):843–852.

Armengol CE, Hendley O, Schlager TA. Should we abandon standard microscopy when screening for urinary tract infections in young children? *Pediatr Infect Dis J* 2001;20(12):1176–117.

Hoberman A, Wald ER, Reynolds EA, et al. Is urine culture necessary to rule out urinary tract infection in young febrile children. *Pediatr Infect Dis J* 1996;15(4):304–309.

McDonald A, Scranton M, Gillespie R, et al. Voiding cystourethrogram and urinary tract infections: how long to wait? *Pediatrics* 2000;105(4): E50.

11

Meningitis

Meningitis is defined as inflammation of the meninges. The term meningitis denotes only the presence of inflammation and not a specific etiology. The specific etiology of meningitis is determined by clinical history, cerebrospinal fluid (CSF) profile, cultures, and specific studies of the CSF.

BACTERIAL MENINGITIS

Epidemiology

Bacterial meningitis is the most feared form of pediatric meningitis. Bacteria, which colonize the skin, nasopharynx, or both, enter the bloodstream. These bacteria then "seed" the CSF. It is for this reason that blood cultures are positive in up to 90% of children with bacterial meningitis.

Presentation

Patients with bacterial meningitis typically present with high fevers, headache, and an altered mental state. The classic clinical triad of bacterial meningitis is fever, nuchal rigidity, and a change in mental status, although only two thirds of patients with bacterial meningitis actually have all three of these symptoms. Kernig's sign is a clinical examination technique whereby 90% flexion of the hips causes subsequent painful extension of the legs. Brudzinski's sign is involuntary flexion of the knees and hips after passive flexion of the neck while supine. Although these clinical signs have traditionally been used to evaluate for bacterial meningitis, recent studies in adults have found that Kernig's and Brudzinski's signs actually have a low sensitivity for predicting the presence of bacterial meningitis. The entire clinical picture should be used in determining whether to obtain a lumbar puncture.

Diagnosis

The major reported risk in obtaining a sample of CSF is that a preexisting intracranial mass will cause a brainstem herniation following lumbar puncture. There are also concerns that lumbar puncture could cause herniation in a child who has increased intracranial pressure secondary to severe meningitis. Many clinicians obtain a computed tomography (CT) scan of the head before obtaining a lumbar puncture, although this may delay diagnosis and optimal therapy. Although herniation remains a possibility in the setting of bacterial meningitis, it remains an uncommon occurrence, with most estimates reporting an incidence of less than 5%. Although an increase in intracranial pressure is thought to be present in virtually all cases of pediatric bacterial meningitis, it is also known that CT of the brain is normal in most cases of bacterial meningitis, including cases that had subsequent herniation following lumbar puncture. Most specialists stress the need for an accurate history and physical examination when deciding whether to obtain imaging before lumbar puncture. It is noted that a patient with a mass lesion such as an abscess or brain tumor will usually report symptoms over the preceding weeks, whereas in bacterial meningitis, there is a history ranging from hours to days. The diagnosis of impending cerebral herniation can often be made clinically from abnormalities of the neurological exam, including sixth nerve palsy, dilated or fixed pupils, and decerebrate posturing. In patients who have the clinical features of impending herniation, lumbar puncture should be deferred and diagnostic testing limited to blood cultures. Aggressive measures to reduce intracranial pressure are mandatory in such a patient.

Cerebrospinal Fluid Examination

Examination of the CSF is critical. Typically, bacterial meningitis presents with a CSF white blood cell count of several thousand white cells, most being segmented neutrophils. The mean CSF white cell count in bacterial meningitis, regardless of whether patients have been pretreated, is greater than $4,000/m^3$. In bacterial meningitis, the protein concentration of the CSF will be high and glucose concentration low. The probability of a positive Gram stain is dependent on the number of bacteria present in the CSF, which may be related to the timing of lumbar puncture in relation to the onset of symptoms. A positive Gram stain of the CSF in bacterial meningitis is also related to the organism causing the meningitis. *Streptococcus pneumoniae* has the highest rate of having a positive Gram stain (about 90%), with *Neisseria meningitidis* having a positive Gram stain in about 75% of cases. CSF cultures are more likely to be positive in patients who had lumbar puncture before the administration of antibiotics.

Management

Empiric Therapy for Bacterial Meningitis

When faced with a patient with presumed bacterial meningitis, it is optimal to start appropriate antibiotics as early as possible. The "Gram stain game" can help in this decision. The following are the major pathogens of pediatric bacterial meningitis.

1. ***Streptococcus agalactiae*: group B streptococcus.** A gram-positive coccus, group B streptococcus is a common cause of neonatal meningitis. Up to one half of women are colonized with *S. agalactiae* in the genital tract; neonates become colonized at the time of delivery. A certain percentage of these neonates then become bacteremic, which can result in CSF infection. Therapy is with ampicillin and gentamicin.

2. ***Streptococcus pneumoniae*.** Another gram-positive coccus, this is the most common cause of infant and toddler meningitis. The mechanism is similar to that of group B streptococcus, whereby colonizing bacteria entering the bloodstream with subsequent infection of the CSF.

3. ***Neisseria meningitidis*.** A gram-negative diplococcus, this can cause rapid onset of meningitis, septic shock, and death. Septic shock associated with *N. meningitidis* is often associated with rapid onset of petechial and purpuric lesions. Therapy is with a third-generation cephalosporin or intravenous penicillin.

4. ***Listeria monocytogenes*.** A gram-positive rod, this organism is ubiquitous in the environment and commonly found in unpasteurized food products. Meningitis usually occurs in the neonatal period and in immunocompromised patients. This is the one cause of bacterial meningitis not sensitive to the third-generation cephalosporins. Ampicillin is the drug of choice, used in combination with gentamycin. For patients who cannot tolerate ampicillin, intravenous trimethoprim-sulfamethoxazole is recommended as the second choice. Vancomycin may be a successful alternative antibiotic, although treatment failures have also been reported.

5. ***Haemophilus influenzae* (type b).** Before the development of the conjugate vaccine, this gram-negative coccobacillus frequently caused invasive disease. Pediatricians rarely encounter type b *H. influenzae* meningitis in unvaccinated populations. There are increasing reports of nontypeable *Haemophilus* causing invasive disease, including meningitis. Treatment is with a third-generation cephalosporin; ampicillin can be used if the causative bacteria are β-lactamase negative.

Pathogen	Comments	Antibiotics
Neisseria meningitidis	Gram-negative diplococcus Associated with purpura fulminans	1. Penicillin G, 100,000–400,000 units/kg per day in four divided doses 2. Ceftriaxone, 100 mg/kg per day in two divided doses 3. Cefotaxime, 200 mg/kg per day in three divided doses
Haemophilus influenzae (type b)	Gram-negative coccobacillus	1. Third-generation cephalosporin, or ampicillin if β-lactamase negative
Listeria monocytogenes	Gram-positive rod Occurs in neonates, immunocompromised patients	1. Ampicillin, 200–400 mg/kg per day in four divided doses 2. Gentamicin, 6–7.5 mg/kg per day in three divided doses

Special Considerations: Treatment of Streptococcus pneumoniae

The most common cause of infant and toddler meningitis remains *S. pneumoniae*, although this may ultimately change owing to the recent addition of the conjugate vaccine to primary immunization series.

Resistance of *S. pneumoniae*. One of the major issues in the treatment of pneumococcal meningitis is the increasing resistance to penicillin and cephalosporins. Resistance is mediated by alterations in penicillin-binding proteins. This increases the minimal inhibitory concentration (MIC) to both these antibiotics; that is, increased concentrations of antibiotic are needed to inhibit growth of bacteria. The problem faced with treating meningitis in the context of increasing MIC is as follows:

1. A CSF antibiotic concentration of 10 times the MIC of the infecting organism is required to ensure cure in an infection as serious as meningitis.
2. Because of the blood–brain barrier, there is a limit to antibiotic concentration achievable in the CSF. As MIC values increase, a CSF antibiotic concentration of 10 times the MIC cannot be achieved.

The **breakpoint** is the highest MIC at which an organism is defined as sensitive to a given drug. The desire to achieve a CSF concentration of 10 times the MIC explains the breakpoints for penicillin and third-generation cephalosporins for the treatment of *S. pneumoniae* meningitis. The maximal concentration of penicillin obtained in the CSF is about 1.0 µg/mL. The breakpoint for the use of penicillin in pneumococcal meningitis is 0.06 µg/mL; any MIC to penicillin of an infecting pneumococcus greater than this does not guarantee a concentration 10 times the MIC. The maximal concentration for a third-generation cephalosporin in the CSF is about 5.0 µg/mL. The breakpoint for cefotaxime or ceftriaxone is 0.5 µg/mL; if the MIC is greater than 0.5, a concentration in the spinal fluid of 10 times the MIC cannot be ensured.

Rates of resistance vary from community to community. Rates of *S. pneumoniae* with an MIC to penicillin greater than 0.1 µg/mL can be as high as 75%. Rates of pneumococcus with an MIC to a third-generation cephalosporin greater than 0.5 µg/mL can approach 20%. These numbers may increase as antibiotic overuse persists. It is for this reason that empiric therapy for presumed pneumococcal meningitis includes vancomycin (15 mg/kg given intravenously every 6 hours) and a third-generation cephalosporin. All pneumococcal isolates from the CSF should be tested for MIC to penicillin and third-generation cephalosporins. After specific MICs are available, therapy can be tailored appropriately.

There is little experience, although justifiable concern, in the management of children with pneumococcal meningitis in which the isolated bacteria has an MIC to cefotaxime or ceftriaxone greater than 2.0 µg/mL. In those cases, treatment with both vancomycin and a third-generation cephalosporin is recommended. The addition of rifampin, 20 mg/kg in two divided doses, should also be considered.

Meropenem is a new antibiotic that has excellent gram-negative coverage and good CSF penetration. Although approved for children 3 months of age or older with penicillin-susceptible pneumococcal meningitis, there is little clinical experience with this drug in resistant pneumococcal isolates. In the coming years, more data regarding meropenem in the treatment of resistant pneumococcal meningitis will be available.

Antibiotic Therapy for Streptococcus pneumoniae Meningitis

- Penicillin susceptible (MIC < 0.1μg/mL)
  Penicillin, 100,000–400,000 units/kg per day in four divided doses
- Penicillin intermediate (MIC = 0.1–1.0 μg/mL)
  Cefotaxime, 200 mg/kg per day in three divided doses
  Ceftriaxone, 100 mg/kg day in two divided doses
- Penicillin resistant (MIC > 1.0 μg/mL)
  Cefotaxime, 200 mg/kg per day in three divided doses
  Ceftriaxone, 100 mg/kg per day in two divided doses
- Cefotaxime or ceftriaxone sensitive (MIC < 0.5 μg/mL)
  Cefotaxime, 200 mg/kg per day in three divided doses
  Ceftriaxone, 100 mg/kg per day in two divided doses
- Cefotaxime or ceftriaxone intermediate (MIC = 0.5–2.0 μg/mL)
  Third-generation cephalosporin with vancomycin, 15 mg/kg every 6 hours
- Cefotaxime or ceftriaxone resistant (MIC > 2.0 μg/mL)
  Third-generation cephalosporin with vancomycin, 15 mg/kg every 6 hours; consider adding rifampin, 20 mg/kg per day. Can also consider meropenem, 120 mg/kg per day in three divided doses

---

Steroid Therapy for Bacterial Meningitis

During the past decade, increasing attention has been given to adjunctive treatment for bacterial meningitis. It is recognized that bacterial meningitis is a disorder of intense inflammation and that this inflammation can result in substantial morbidity, primarily in the form of hearing loss. For patients with *H. influenzae* type B meningitis, dexamethasone is recommended. The dose is 0.15 mg/kg of dexamethasone every 6 hours for 4 days.

The use of steroids in pneumococcal meningitis is more controversial. A major concern is a possible decrease in antibiotic concentration in the CSF when steroids are given. In animal models, vancomycin concentration was altered up to 75% when concurrent steroids were used. The few clinical trials performed have not shown CSF differences in vancomycin and cefotaxime concentrations in the presence of dexamethasone. Two retrospective studies regarding outcome in patients with resistant pneumococcal meningitis receiving dexamethasone have been published, reaching different conclusions. In a small number of children with bacterial meningitis who received both vancomycin and dexamethasone, vancomycin levels in the CSF were comparable to those measured in children who receive vancomycin without dexamethasone. At this point, the opinion of the American Academy of Pediatrics is that the clinician needs to evaluate each case individually, weighing risks and benefits of steroid use.

ASEPTIC MENINGITIS

Etiology

The term **aseptic meningitis** is defined as meningitis associated with negative bacterial cultures. Most cases of aseptic meningitis are caused by viral pathogens, with enterovirus being the leading cause. Enteroviruses comprise several serotypes, including coxsackievirus, echovirus, and poliovirus. These pathogens predominate in the summer or fall months and may cause epidemics of disease.

Presentation

Patients usually present with acute onset of fever, headache, and vomiting. Clinical signs of meningeal irritation may be present. Photophobia and myalgias are common. There may be an associated gastroenteritis. Patients are typically not as acutely ill as those with bacterial meningitis.

Evaluation of Cerebrospinal Fluid

A common challenge facing the pediatrician is using the results of the CSF to determine whether the child has aseptic meningitis. Aseptic meningitis is typically characterized by a few hundred white blood cells, most of which are lymphocytes. In contrast, bacterial meningitis is characterized by thousands of white blood cells with a segmented neutrophil predominance. It also should be noted that in most cases of bacterial meningitis, there are other abnormalities seen in the CSF, such as a positive Gram stain and low glucose and high protein levels.

Standard textbooks also state that aseptic meningitis can have a predominance of polymorphonuclear cells early in the course of disease. It has long been thought that in aseptic meningitis with an early segmented neutrophil predominance, repeat lumbar puncture after 24 hours will document the typical picture of lymphocytic predominance. Recent studies have challenged this assumption; one study showed that most children with aseptic meningitis in the height of the enteroviral season actually maintained a predominance of segmented neutrophils in the CSF even after the first 24 hours of illness. These same studies also pointed out that the average number of white blood cells in patients with viral meningitis remains in the low 100s, whereas in bacterial meningitis, it is several thousand. Ultimately, the clinician evaluating the CSF from a patient will need to consider the entire clinical picture, including history, clinical exam, and abnormalities of the spinal fluid.

Diagnosis

Enterovirus can be cultured from CSF. Polymerase chain reaction (PCR) has been shown to be more sensitive than culture, and in many settings, results can be available in less than 24 hours.

Management

Treatment is generally supportive, including hydration and pain management.

ENCEPHALITIS

> **Encephalitis** refers to inflammation of the brain. Meningoencephalitis is a condition in which both brain and meninges are affected.

Etiology

Encephalitis can be caused by any of a long list of infectious agents. These pathogens can cause encephalitis by either direct invasion of the brain or by a postinflammatory effect. The exact mechanisms for certain agents are not well defined.

Determining the etiology of a particular encephalitis can be challenging. Brain biopsy is usually not performed. Many pathogens causing encephalitis are fastidious and are difficult to grow in standard culture. Serology has historically been a mainstay of diagnosis; recent advances in PCR technology have been employed to maximize yield in the diagnosis of encephalitis.

Presentation

Patients with encephalitis usually are sicker than those with typical aseptic meningitis because the brain itself is inflamed. Seizures are common, as are focal neurologic deficits and cognitive disturbances. CSF often shows an "aseptic" picture with several hundred white blood cells, most of which are lymphocytes.

The following is a brief discussion of the major pathogens implicated in pediatric encephalitis. In evaluating a patient with encephalitis, a complete history, particularly in regard to travel, animal exposure, concurrent immunosuppression, and geographic location, is critical.

Herpes Simplex Virus

Epidemiology and Etiology

Herpes simplex virus (HSV) is responsible for up to 30% of diagnosed adult viral encephalitis. Infection is thought to begin with colonization or infection in the nasopharynx; invasive disease can then result because HSV has an affinity for the frontal and temporal lobes of the brain.

Presentation

The clinical spectrum of herpes simplex encephalitis has been reevaluated as diagnostic testing has become more sensitive. Once thought to be primarily a cause of acute encephalitis, it is appreciated that a more chronic course, including febrile seizures and progressive loss of higher cognitive function, is possible. The focal hemorrhagic nature of herpes encephalitis is well described. Younger patients are more likely to have characteristic lesions in areas other than the temporal lobes typically described in adults. Seizures are common, and progression to coma is frequently seen.

Diagnosis

The diagnosis of herpes simplex involves several techniques. Electroencephalography is a noninvasive technique that shows temporal lobe spikes in about 80% of cases. Viral culture of the CSF is not very sensitive, resulting in positive cultures in only 20% of cases. PCR of the spinal fluid is considered to be the new gold standard for diagnosis of herpes simplex encephalitis. Although PCR of spinal fluid offers an improvement over previous diagnostic techniques, caution should be employed. Recent studies have shown that young children may have negative PCR in CSF, especially if CSF is sampled on the first or second day of illness. It has been postulated that early in HSV encephalitis, the virus is in the brain but is absent from the CSF. Evaluation for herpes simplex encephalitis in young children should take into account the entire clinical picture, particularly if characteristic lesions are seen on neuroimaging. In certain cases in which the clinical picture is consistent with herpes simplex encephalitis, a second CSF sample should be obtained. Antiviral therapy will have little effect on the presence of HSV DNA in the CSF; prior administration of acyclovir should not preclude the continuing evaluation for herpes simplex in the CSF.

Management

HSV is one of the few treatable forms of encephalitis. Many infectious disease specialists believe that encephalitis is herpes simplex until proved otherwise. Patients with a clinical picture of meningoencephalitis should be started on acyclovir at a dose of 10 mg/kg every 8 hours.

Enteroviruses

Epidemiology and Etiology

Enteroviruses are in the family Picornaviridae, which includes poliovirus, coxsackie, and echovirus. These are a major cause of both pediatric aseptic meningitis and encephalitis. Epidemics of nonpolio enteroviral infections frequently occur in late summer and early fall.

Presentation

Children with enteroviral encephalitis initially may have fever, headache, and photophobia, often accompanied by symptoms of gastroenteritis. Encephalitis will then manifest with seizures, focal neurologic deficits, and altered mental status. Neonates with enteroviral disease may have a disseminated illness that closely resembles that caused by herpes simplex virus. These neonates in the first weeks of life may present with fever, liver failure, and coagulopathy.

Diagnosis

Diagnosis of enteroviral disease is as described previously. PCR can be obtained on serum and CSF and is the quickest and most sensitive diagnostic test.

Management

Treatment is generally supportive. Pleconaril is an oral antiviral agent that has been shown in compassionate use trials to be effective in some cases of severe disease, including disseminated neonatal disease.

Mycoplasma pneumoniae

Epidemiology and Etiology

M. pneumoniae is a common respiratory pathogen that is thought to be a major cause of pediatric encephalitis. In some series, it is the leading identifiable cause of encephalitis in children.

The organism has been isolated from brain and CSF by culture and PCR. Isolation implies direct invasion of the pathogen, although *M. pneumoniae* has also been implicated as a cause of immune-mediated disease, such as acute demyelinating encephalopathy, Guillain-Barré syndrome, and transverse myelitis. The mechanism of immune-mediated disease is proposed antigenic similarities between *M. pneumoniae* and human neural tissue. It is speculated that patients with shorter prodromes may have a direct-invasion disease mechanism, whereas those with longer prodromes may have immune-mediated disease.

Presentation

Prodromal respiratory illness lasting days to weeks occurs in some patients, although disease has been documented without preceding respiratory symptoms. Mycoplasma encephalitis can be associated with focal neurologic signs thought to be the result of associated acute demyelination.

Diagnosis

The diagnosis of *M. pneumoniae* encephalitis is by culture, PCR of the CSF, or both. Serology can also be used, although false-negative results can occur.

Management

Treatment is supportive. A variety of treatments, including antibiotics intravenous immune globulin and corticosteroids, have been attempted, although there is no definite consensus as to their use.

Pediatric Viral Infections

A large number of common pediatric viral infections have been reportedly associated with encephalitis. These include Epstein-Barr virus, influenza virus, and cytomegalovirus. The mechanism of the encephalitis is not known, being either direct viral invasion or secondary immune response. In the setting of encephalitis, serologies for these pathogens, as well as PCR studies, can be useful in diagnoses.

ARBOVIRUSES

Arboviruses are arthropod-borne viruses spread by mosquitos, ticks, or sand flies. These pathogens cause a wide spectrum of illness ranging from self-limited febrile illnesses to aseptic meningitis to encephalitis. Certain arboviruses are present in specific regions in the United States and usually occur in late summer and early autumn.

California encephalitis (La Crosse Virus)

Etiology

La Crosse encephalitis is caused by Bunyavirus. The name is a misnomer, reflecting not geographic location but rather the initial place of discovery. The disease is actually found in the Midwestern and Eastern United States. It is often considered the most common pediatric arboviral infection in the United States.

Presentation

There is a spectrum of disease from mild febrile illness to aseptic meningitis to fatal encephalitis. There is usually a febrile prodrome, which can include headache and vomiting. La Crosse encephalitis occurs mostly in children; seizures are the presenting symptom in one half of cases. Focal neurologic signs, including paralysis, are seen in one fourth of cases.

Diagnosis

Diagnosis is by serologic methods, usually an immunoglobulin M (IgM) enzyme-linked immunosorbent assay (ELISA) capture antibody.

Management

Treatment is supportive. Ribavirin has been used in clinical trials, although no definitive proof of its usefulness exists.

St. Louis Encephalitis

Etiology

St. Louis encephalitis is caused by a virus in the Flaviviridae family. This is considered an important arboviral infection due to its ability to cause epidemics of disease. A large number of cases have been reported in midwestern states as well as in Texas, Louisiana, and Florida.

Presentation

Patients with St. Louis encephalitis often present with headache and fever. Associated paralysis or weakness can occur, as can multiple cranial nerve palsies.

Diagnosis

Diagnosis is by serology, usually IgM ELISA.

Management

Treatment is supportive. No specific medical therapy is currently available.

West Nile Virus

Etiology

West Nile virus is the arbovirus most reported in the medical news. It appeared in North America in 1999 in New York City, causing 62 cases, with seven deaths. A flavivirus found commonly along major bird migration pathways, it is transmitted to birds by mosquitos, which can also infect humans. Transmission through organ transplantation, blood transfusion, and breast milk has also been reported.

Presentation

Most infections are asymptomatic; infection can also be a self-limited febrile illness sometimes accompanied by a transient rash. Less than 1% of infections result in encephalitis. Extremes of age appear to be a risk factor for encephalitis. Patients with central nervous system involvement can exhibit encephalitis, abnormalities of movement, and ocular motor dysfunction. Examination of the CSF shows pleocytosis, with the majority of cells being mononuclear. Early signs of more severe neurologic disease include Guillain-Barré syndrome and transverse myelitis and can provide a clue to diagnosis.

Diagnosis

Diagnosis of West Nile virus is made primarily by serology. ELISA or immunofluorescent assay (IFA) are frequently used. PCR assays are also becoming available. Viremia, as detected by PCR, can be found before the onset of symptoms.

Management

There is no specific therapy for West Nile virus encephalitis. Ribavirin has been shown to inhibit the virus in neural cell cultures and has been administered to a small number of patients. There is no consensus on treatment. The major role of medical treatment remains supportive care (Table 11.1).

TABLE 11.1. *Evaluation of Cerebrospinal Fluid in Pediatric Encephalitis*

Pathogen	Diagnosis
1. Herpes simplex	a. CSF viral culture
	b. PCR, CSF
	c. EEG reveals temporal lobe spikes in 80%
2. Enteroviruses	a. Viral culture, CSF
	b. Polymerase chain reaction, CSF
	c. Viral culture of nasopharynx and stool (suggestive, not diagnostic)
3. *Mycoplasma pneumoniae*	a. Serology for mycoplasma IgM, IgG
	b. PCR in cerebrospinal fluid
4. Arbovirus	a. Serology
a. West Nile virus	
b. California equine (La Crosse)	
c St. Louis	

CSF, cerebrospinal fluid; PCR, polymerase chain reaction; EEG, electroencephalogram; Ig, immunoglobulin.

FUNGAL MENINGITIS

Fungal meningitis is usually, but not exclusively, seen in patients with underlying immunodeficiency. The major organisms to be considered include *Coccidioides immitis* and *Cryptococcus neoformans*.

Coccidioides immitis Infection

Etiology

This dysmorphic fungus is found in soil and infects people through inhalation of airborne spores.

Presentation

The most common manifestation in the normal host is a self-limited bronchitis. Disseminated disease occurs in less than 1% of infections, with the bones, skin, and central nervous system being common secondary sites. Severe disease is frequent in patients with underlying T-cell immunodeficiency, such as those infected with the human immunodeficiency virus (HIV). It can also be found in normal hosts, with African-American and Filipino patients at higher risk for disseminated disease.

In the immunocompetent host, the cerebrospinal profile is similar to a viral meningitis with several hundred cells, most of which are lymphocytes. In the severely immunocompromised patient, there may not be adequate functioning lymphocytes to cause an appropriate inflammatory response. In these patients, there may be a normal CSF even in the face of a severe fungal meningitis.

Diagnosis

Complement fixation antibodies in the serum and CSF are often used to make the diagnosis. Increasing antibody titers indicate progressive disease. Fungal cultures of CSF can also be used for the diagnosis.

Management

Treatment is always indicated for coccidioidomycosis meningitis. Treatment of coccidioidomycosis meningitis is usually with oral fluconazole, which achieves good levels in the CSF. Dosage is 400 mg per day, although doses as high as 1 g per day have been used. As with any granulomatous meningitis, hydrocephalus secondary to obstruction of cerebrospinal flow is always a possibility. If this complication develops, a ventriculoperitoneal shunt may be required. Therapy is typically indefinite in patients with CNS infection because withdrawing of medication often results in relapsed infection.

Cryptococcus neoformans Infection

Etiology

The etiology of *C. neoformans* meningitis is similar to that of coccidioidomycosis; it is found in soil contaminated with bird droppings and causes infection through inhalation of the organism.

Presentation

In patients with HIV infection, it is one of the most common causes of central nervous system infection. These patients present with a severe headache but can also present with behavioral changes or focal neurologic signs.

Diagnosis

In patients with underlying immunodeficiency, the CSF may not contain numerous lymphocytes. Encapsulated yeast can be visualized by India ink staining of the spinal fluid. Antigen detection against the capsular polysaccharide of the organism in CSF is positive in more than 90% of patients. The organism can also be grown in fungal culture.

Management

Treatment of cryptococcal meningitis is with amphotericin B in doses of 0.5 to 0.7 mg/kg per day in combination with oral flucytosine (5-FC). When flucytosine is used, serum concentration should be monitored, as should complete blood counts. Patients should continue combination therapy for at least 2 weeks or until repeat culture of the CSF is negative. Immunocompromised patients with cryptococcal meningitis, as in patients with *C. immitis* meningitis, typically receive lifelong maintenance therapy with fluconazole.

SELECTED READINGS

De Tiège X, Heron B, Lebon P, et al. Limits of early diagnosis of herpes simplex encephalitis in children: a retrospective study of 38 Cases. *Clin Infect Dis* 2003;36(10):1335–1339.

Glaser CA, Gilliam S, Schnurr D, et al. In search of encephalitis etiologies: diagnostic challenges in the California Encephalitis Project 1998–2000. *Clin Infect Dis* 2003;36(6):731–742.

Greenlee JE. Approach to diagnosis of meningitis. Cerebrospinal fluid evaluation. *Infect Dis Clin North Am* 1990;4(4):583–598.

Oliver WJ, Shope TC, Kuhns LR. Fatal lumbar puncture: fact verus fiction. An approach to a clinical dilemma. *Pediatrics* 2003;112(3):3 174–176.

12

Pediatric Tuberculosis

EPIDEMIOLOGY

After years of decline in the national rates of tuberculosis, there were discussions in the early 1980s regarding the elimination of the disease in the United States. However, from the mid-1980s to the early 1990s, there was a 15% increase in reported cases. Children were even more greatly affected by this trend, with an increase in reported cases in children 5 to 14 years of age of almost 40%. The increase in cases of tuberculosis was thought to be the result of an increase in medically underserved populations, an increased number of patients from endemic areas, and an increase in patients infected with human immunodeficiency virus (HIV) resulting in large numbers of contagious patients. Although infection control efforts have been somewhat successful in controlling tuberculosis, it remains a major cause of morbidity and mortality in selected areas of the United States. This chapter discusses both the pathophysiology of pediatric tuberculous infection and the diagnosis and therapy of latent and active disease.

ETIOLOGY

Infection with *Mycobacterium tuberculosis* (MTB) begins with the inhalation of airborne bacilli. After inhalation, the bacilli reach the pulmonary alveoli and are transported through pulmonary lymphatic channels to hilar lymph nodes. They can then enter the bloodstream by way of the thoracic duct. Although the entrance of MTB into the host is respiratory, the organism can thus be spread to virtually every organ in the body. Spread of small numbers of bacilli result in clinically inapparent foci of infection. Regions most commonly seeded include the meninges, the pleura, and the bone. A reaction involving macrophages, lymphocytes, and ingested organisms then occurs, and tubercles are formed. When this reaction occurs, a tuberculin skin test will become positive, indicating that exposure to MTB has occurred.

The initial immune containment of clinically inapparent infection may not be permanent, and reactivation is possible at any time. Infants younger than 1 year of age have about a 50% chance of developing active disease. In children younger than 5 years of age, the risk for reactivation to active disease is about 25%.

PRESENTATION OF LATENT TUBERCULOSIS

A child who is infected with MTB without clinical or radiographic signs is defined as having latent infection. There is a great advantage in diagnosing and treating latent infection because it can avoid subsequent reactivation and the development of active disease.

DIAGNOSIS

Tuberculin skin testing (TST) is the method used for diagnosing latent infection. The TST used is the Mantoux test, containing five tuberculin units administered intradermally. This test is read as millimeters of induration at 48 to 72 hours.

The definition of a positive TST is based on a variety of epidemiologic and clinical factors. Induration of greater than 15 mm is considered positive in children older than 4 years of age without specific risk factors. A TST of greater than or equal to 10 mm is positive in children younger than 4 years of age and in children with other medical conditions, including renal failure, diabetes, or malignancy. This is also considered positive in children with increased risk for exposure, including those residing in areas with a high prevalence of tuberculosis. An induration of greater than 5 mm is considered positive in children receiving immunosuppressive therapy or with underlying immunodeficiency conditions. This induration is also considered positive if one has close contact with a case of active tuberculosis or has clinical or radiographic evidence of the disease (Table 12.1).

Use of Anergy Testing

Up to 20% of patients with active tuberculosis have a negative TST at initial presentation. In the 1970s, the idea of evaluating negative tuberculin tests results by assessing reactions to a panel of unrelated antigens (such as candida or tetanus) was proposed. This concept of **anergy testing** became a routine adjunct to tuberculin

TABLE 12.1. *Criteria for Positive Tuberculin Skin Test*

Reaction	Population
1. Greater than 5-mm induration	1. Human immunodeficiency virus (HIV) positive
	2. Radiographic evidence of tuberculosis
	3. Contacts of contagious patients
	4. Immunosuppressive individuals including organ transplantation and/or patients receiving $\geq$ 15 mg/d prednisone
2. Greater than 10-mm induration	1. Children younger than 4 yrs
	2. Recent immigrants (i.e., within past 5 yrs) from high-prevalence countries
	3. Residents of high-risk settings including nursing homes, jails, homeless shelters
3. Greater than 15-mm induration	1. Persons with no risk factors for tuberculosis
	2. Children older than 4 yrs

skin testing. Despite its widespread use, the validity of this approach has never been proved. The ability to respond to other antigens has been shown not to improve the reliability of a negative TST test. Studies have also shown that the results of anergy testing do not predict the risk for progression to active disease in either HIV-negative or HIV-positive patients. For this reason, routine anergy testing, used as a validation to tuberculin skin testing, is not recommended by most infectious disease specialists.

Although Bacille Calmette-Guérin (BCG) vaccine is not routinely given in the United States, the pediatrician will need to interpret TST in children who have received this vaccine. After BCG vaccination, distinguishing a positive reaction secondary to latent infection from reactivity to BCG is difficult. One study found that only 8% of persons who had received BCG vaccine at birth had a positive TST 15 years later. It is for this reason that the American Academy of Pediatrics recommends the same criteria for TST interpretation in patients who have received BCG.

Booster Phenomenon

Reactivity from TST resulting from MTB exposure may actually decrease over time in some patients, resulting in a nonreactive test despite a history of past exposure and latent infection. In these cases, the stimulus of a tuberculin test may actually "boost" or increase the size of any subsequent TST. This positive TST may be misleading because it may suggest recent tuberculin conversion when in fact latent infection has been present for years. Adults who undergo annual TST, particularly health care workers, often undergo two-step testing on initial evaluation with a second TST administered 1 week after the initial test. In this way, the boosting phenomenon can be appropriately evaluated and not mistaken for a recent skin test conversion.

Management of Latent Infection

Children who have a positive TST require a chest x-ray. In children younger than 18 years of age with a positive TST and negative chest x-ray, the diagnosis of latent tuberculous infection is made. Monotherapy is acceptable only in the case of latent tuberculosis infection. Patients younger than 18 years of age who have latent infection with an isoniazid-sensitive organism are treated with isoniazid for 9 months. Latent infection with an isoniazid-resistant organism is treated with a 6-month course of oral rifampin. Children younger than 5 years of age have a very high risk for severe tuberculosis when exposed to a contagious index case. Even if such a child's first TST is negative, it is recommended that antituberculosis medication be given. Medication can then be discontinued if a second TST 3 months later remains negative and the child has no clinical signs of tuberculosis.

Previously, the Centers for Disease Control (CDC) recommended prophylaxis with pyrazinamide and ethambutol for patients exposed to isoniazid- and rifampin-resistant mycobacteria. Surveillance done by the CDC has reported numerous cases of severe liver injury in patients receiving this prophylaxis. The updated recommendation is for clinicians to practice extreme caution in treating latent infection with the combination of pyrazinamide and ethambutol, especially if there are risk factors for liver injury, including concurrent hepatotoxic medications or alcohol consumption. Patients who elect to take this regimen should be followed closely, both clinically and with frequent measurement of serum aminotransferase levels.

ACTIVE TUBERCULOUS INFECTION

In a percentage of cases after exposure to MTB, the latent tuberculous infection can reactivate. At this point, the child is considered to have active tuberculous infection. It is important to note that there are a variety of clinical syndromes associated with active disease.

Common Clinical Manifestations of Active Pediatric Tuberculosis

- Pulmonary disease
- Miliary disease
- Meningitis
- Pleural effusion

TUBERCULOUS PNEUMONIA

Epidemiology

The most common clinical manifestation of active pediatric tuberculous disease is pulmonary tuberculosis. Unlike adults who present with cavitary disease, pediatric pulmonary tuberculosis usually presents as hilar adenopathy.

Presentation

The hilar enlargement of pulmonary tuberculosis typically produces little or no symptoms in older children; up to 80% of children older than 5 years of age are asymptomatic. Unlike older children, infants with hilar adenopathy may become symptomatic. The smaller caliber of bronchi in infants is more easily compressed by the enlarging lymph nodes, and the progressive lymphadenopathy can cause obstruction with resultant air trapping and wheezing (Figs. 12.1 and 12.2).

Diagnosis

The diagnosis of pulmonary tuberculosis in the child often rests on a positive TST and a chest radiograph that shows pulmonary disease. Therefore, accurate radiographic diagnosis is crucial for correct diagnosis of pediatric pulmonary tu-

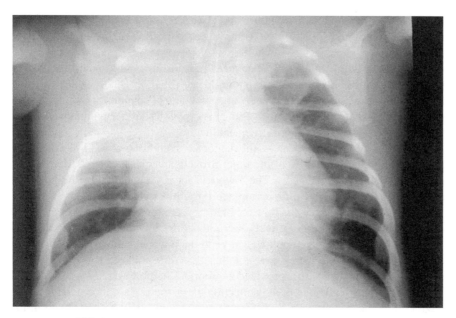

FIG. 12.1. Large hilar adenopathy seen in child with tuberculosis.

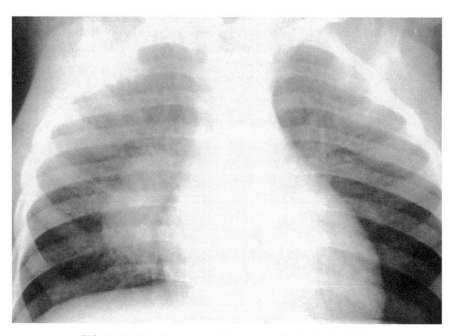

FIG. 12.2. Early hilar adenopathy representing typical pediatric
pulmonary tuberculosis.

berculosis. When there is uncertainty about whether hilar adenopathy is present, computed tomography (CT) has been shown to be helpful in confirming the diagnosis.

Isolation of MTB from clinical specimens remains the gold standard for diagnosis. Isolation of MTB in children is more difficult than in adults, who frequently have cavitary disease and can produce large amounts of sputum for culture. An aggressive workup aimed at isolation of infective mycobacteria should always be attempted because this will guide subsequent therapy.

Even in tertiary medical centers, the diagnosis in children of MTB is confirmed by culture no more than 40% of the time. Bronchoalveolar lavage (BAL) yields a pathogen in about 20% of cases. The low yield for BAL is likely due to the specimen collected over a brief time period and only in selected pulmonary segments. The fact that children often swallow respiratory secretions can be used in the isolation of MTB. Gastric lavage of early-morning stomach contents contains material collected over an entire evening and can yield the positive culture in up to 50% of cases. A recent study also suggested that this procedure could be successfully done during serial outpatient visits, provided appropriate support systems were in place. The use of proper technique in the collection of gastric aspirate is crucial in maximizing the yield of this procedure. Gastric aspiration should be performed in the early morning when the patient has been without food for at least 8 hours. Stomach contents are aspirated first through an 8 French feeding tube. Following this, 30 mL of sterile water (not saline) is placed into the stomach and then removed and added to the first collection. Gastric pH should be neutralized within 30 minutes because MTB does not tolerate acid environments. Gastric pH is typically neutralized with a 10% sodium bicarbonate solution. Specimens need to be refrigerated and transported within 4 hours of collection.

Pulmonary Manifestations of Tuberculosis

1. Hilar adenopathy is the most common manifestation.
2. CT can help in the diagnosis.
3. Gastric aspirate and BAL cultures.

MILIARY TUBERCULOSIS

Epidemiology

Miliary tuberculosis represents one of the most severe manifestations of tuberculosis. It represents unchecked dissemination of bacilli to secondary sites, including the liver, brain, and bones.

Presentation

Fever, poor weight gain, and increased respiratory rate are common presenting signs of miliary tuberculosis. Patients with miliary disease may also have diffuse lymphadenopathy and organomegaly.

Diagnosis

Appearance of too-numerous-to-count nodules in the chest x-ray suggests miliary tuberculosis. The nodules may be visualized on CT of the brain even in the absence of cerebrospinal pleocytosis. It is important to realize that, in the setting of an ineffective immune response to tuberculosis, skin testing is frequently negative in miliary disease (Figs. 12.3 and 12.4).

In the setting of miliary disease, cultures bronchoscopy and gastric aspirate are often positive. Biopsy samples of affected organ sites, such as liver, lung, or bone marrow, can also yield the organism.

Miliary Tuberculosis

1. Presentation may include fever, weight loss, or organomegaly.
2. Initial TST may be negative.
3. Central nervous system can be involved without meningitis.
4. Steroids may be helpful if hypoxia is present.

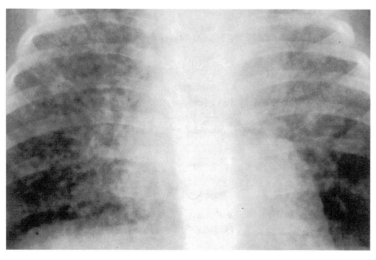

FIG. 12.3. Chest radiograph showing too numerous to count lesions seen in military tuberculosis.

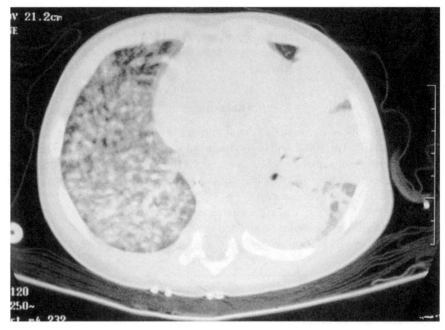

FIG. 12.4. Computed tomograph of the chest in a child with military tuberculosis.

TUBERCULOUS MENINGITIS

Etiology

Tuberculosis meningitis arises from hematogenous dissemination that forms tubercles in the brainstem. After reactivation, these foci may rupture, discharging bacilli into the spinal fluid. A thick exudate subsequently develops, which then impedes the flow of cerebrospinal fluid (CSF).

Presentation

A typical history for tuberculous meningitis is one of progressive lethargy and vomiting over several weeks as hydrocephalus develops and intracranial pressure increases. The chronicity of tuberculosis meningitis helps distinguish it from the more common self-limited pediatric illnesses, such as viral meningitis or gastroenteritis.

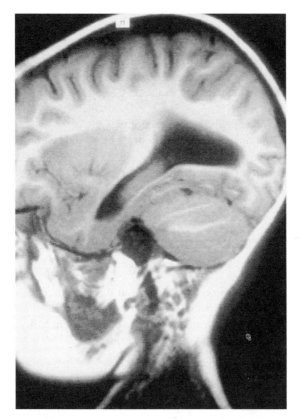

FIG. 12.5. MRI of brain showing hydrocephalous, brainstem inflammation in a child with tuberculosis meningitis.

Diagnosis

In tuberculosis meningitis, CSF examination reveals several hundred cells, most of which are lymphocytes. Cerebrospinal glucose is low, and protein is often elevated. CT of the brain often shows basilar enhancement with hydrocephalus (Fig. 12.5). CT can also be helpful in suggesting the diagnosis because hydrocephalus is a rare occurrence in viral or uncomplicated bacterial meningitis. Acid-fast staining and culture of 1 mL of CSF rarely shows organisms; obtaining a larger volume of up to 15 mL and then cytocentrifuging this larger volume can result in positive acid-fast stain and culture in up to 90% of cases. Although there has been considerable experience in the use of nucleic acid amplification tests for the detection of MTB in respiratory specimens, the use of this technology in CSF is still investigational.

Tuberculous Meningitis

1. Progressive history of lethargy and vomiting indicates increased intracranial pressure.
2. Lymphocytic pleocytosis is found in CSF; profile can resemble viral meningitis.
3. CSF glucose level is low in majority of patients.
4. Chest radiograph is positive in 50% of patients; PPD is positive in 50% of patients.
5. CT reveals hydrocephalus in 80% to 100% of patients.
6. Ventriculoperitoneal shunting is often required.

TUBERCULOUS PLEURAL EFFUSION

Etiology

Tuberculous pleural effusion is secondary to rupture of subpleural foci into the pleural space. The rupture of subpleural foci into the pleural space 6 to 12 weeks after primary infection then promotes a delayed hypersensitivity response to the mycobacterial proteins, resulting in a pleural effusion.

Presentation

Patients can present with fever, cough, and pleuritic pain. Night sweats and hemoptysis are occasionally seen. The chest radiograph often reveals a unilateral pleural effusion (Fig. 12.6). The natural history of tuberculous pleural effusion is complete or significant clearance of the effusion, even without treatment. However, untreated patients have a high rate of developing active pulmonary or extrapulmonary disease within a year. Progression to active disease is greater in young children and immunocompromised patients.

Diagnosis

The diagnosis is suggested in a patient with a unilateral pleural effusion who has a history of exposure to tuberculosis. A one-time thoracentesis is usually indicated because it allows examination of the pleural fluid for diagnostic purposes and can help exclude other etiologies. The pleural fluid usually reveals several hundred cells, most of which are lymphocytes. Less than one third of patients have a positive acid-fast stain or acid-fast culture from pleural fluid. Yield of pleural biopsy is significantly higher and approaches 75%. Adenosine deaminase (ADA) is an enzyme involved in purine catabolism; high levels of ADA have been reported in pleural fluid of patients infected with tuberculosis. Elevated levels of ADA can also be found in patients with an increased number of lymphocytes in the pleural fluid; thus, patients

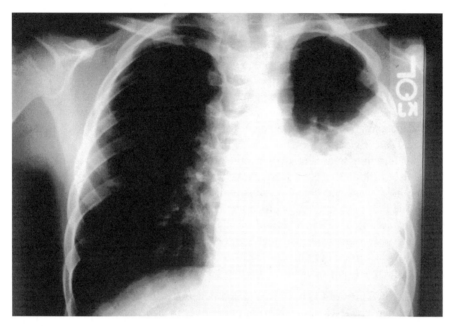

FIG. 12.6. Progressive unilateral pleural effusion seen in child with tuberculosis. Tuberculosis skin test strongly positive.

with leukemias and lymphomas can have misleading results. Polymerase chain reaction for the detection of mycobacterial DNA in pleural effusions is increasingly performed and has a sensitivity of 70% with a specificity of 100%. Most patients with tuberculous pleural effusion have strongly reactive skin tests, and empiric treatment is often given to a patient with a unilateral pleural effusion, a strongly reactive TST, and no other obvious etiology for the effusion.

Pleural Effusion

1. Progressive unilateral effusion is seen with lymphocytic predominance.
2. PPD is often reactive.
3. Natural history is of resolution with high incidence of subsequent pulmonary or extrapulmonary disease.

MANAGEMENT OF ACTIVE PEDIATRIC TUBERCULOSIS

Critical to effective therapy of tuberculosis is the understanding of the presence of naturally occurring mutant organisms within a large population of tuberculous bacilli.

Subpopulations of drug-resistant bacteria are always present within a population of drug-susceptible bacteria. Effective treatment of tuberculosis requires the administration of at least two drugs to which the bacilli is sensitive. If only one effective medication is given, secondary resistance develops within the entire bacilli population.

There was a time when effective two-drug therapy could be guaranteed with the administration of isoniazid and rifampin. The incidence of drug-resistant tuberculous disease continues to increase, largely the result of improper treatment and poor compliance. When initiating treatment for tuberculosis, one can no longer assume isoniazid sensitivity.

When initiating treatment, there should always be an aggressive workup to determine susceptibilities of the infecting mycobacteria. Often, this can be done by finding the index case and obtaining sensitivities on that isolate. This is successful in about one half of cases. If this process is unsuccessful, gastric aspirates and bronchoscopy are often used in an effort to isolate infecting organisms.

In an effort to ensure the use of at least two drugs to which the infecting organism is sensitive, the initial regimen often includes four drugs. The following is a summary of the front-line medications used in pediatric tuberculosis (Table 12.2):

Isoniazid. This drug is bactericidal and penetrates the CSF. Dosage is 10 to 15 mg/kg per day. INH is metabolized in the liver by acetylation. In children, there is no correlation between acetylation efficiency rate and the rate of adverse reaction. The side effects of hepatitis are extremely rare in children. The routine monitoring of liver function tests and vitamin supplementation in patients taking isoniazid alone is not recommended.

Rifampin. This drug is bactericidal and again metabolized by the liver. Dosage is 15 mg/kg per day. Major side effects include orange discoloration of body fluids and interference with oral contraceptives.

Pyrazinamide. This is a well-tolerated drug that penetrates the CSF well. The dose is 20 to 40 mg/kg per day. The major side effects, which are extremely rare, include hepatitis and an increase in uric acid levels.

TABLE 12.2. *Front-line Therapy for Pediatric Tuberculosis*

Drug	Daily dose (mg/kg/d)	Twice weekly dose (mg/kg/dose)	Adverse reactions
Isoniazid	15–25	20–30	a) Hepatitis b) Peripheral neuropathy
Rifampin	10–20	10–20	a) Body secretion discoloration b) Interference with oral contraception
Pyrazinamide	20–40	40–60	a) Hepatitis b) Hyperuricemia
Ethambutol	15	25–50	a) Optic neuritis, decreased red-green color discrimination
Streptomycin (intramuscular)	20–40	20–4—0	a) Nephrotoxicity b) Auditory and vestibular toxicity

Ethambutol. Reports of optic neuritis, which manifests clinically as color blindness, previously precluded use in children because it was thought that children may not be able to verbalize any early visual changes. It has been shown that, at a lower dose of 15 mg/kg per day, the optic neuritis does not occur. Ethambutol is now considered the front-line fourth drug when a fourth drug is indicated.

Duration of Treatment

Using data from thousands of children being treated for tuberculous disease, the American Academy of Pediatrics has issued guidelines for treatment. A 6-month regimen consisting of isoniazid, rifampin, and pyrazinamide for the first 2 months, followed by isoniazid and rifampin for the remaining 4 months, is recommended for the treatment of drug-susceptible pulmonary MTB disease. Extrapulmonary tuberculosis, including meningitis and miliary disease, is generally treated for a total of 12 months.

SELECTED READINGS

Abernathy RS. Tuberculosis: an update. *Pediatr Rev* 1997;18(2):50–8.

Janner D, Rutherford M, Azimi P. Tuberculous meningitis in children. *Pediatr Emerg Care* 1993;9(5): 281–284.

Jasmer RM, Nahid P, Hopewell, PC. Latent tuberculosis infection. *N Engl J Med* 2002;347(23): 1860–1866.

Lobato MN, Loeffler AM, Furst K, et al. Detection of Mycobacterium tuberculosis in gastric aspirates collected from children: hospitalization is not necessary. *Pediatrics* 1998;102(4):E40.

Neu N, Saiman L, San Gabriel P, et al. Diagnosis of pediatric tuberculosis in the modern era. *Pediatr Infect Dis J* 1999;18(2):122–126.

Slovis BS, Plitman JD, Haas DW. The case against anergy testing as a routine adjunct to tuberculin skin testing. *JAMA* 2000;283(15):2003–2007.

13

Community-acquired
Pneumonia

Pediatric lower respiratory infection may be caused by a variety of bacterial and viral pathogens. In addition, the incidence of the atypical pathogens, which include *Mycoplasma pneumoniae, Chlamydia pneumoniae*, and *Legionella pneumophila*, increase as children get older. With such a variety of potential pathogens, clinicians need to develop a method for diagnosing pediatric lower respiratory disease and to differentiate self-limiting viral illness from those caused by bacteria that require specific antibiotic therapy.

EPIDEMIOLOGY

Certain generalizations regarding the etiology of pediatric pneumonia can be made. Viruses cause most lower respiratory diseases in younger children and include respiratory syncytial virus, influenza A and B, parainfluenza, and adenovirus. Respiratory syncytial virus and influenza viruses have their peak incidence in the fall and winter months, whereas parainfluenza dominates in the spring and summer. The presence of wheezing is more common in patients with viral pneumonia as compared with bacterial disease. Bacterial pathogens commonly associated with pneumonia include *Streptococcus pneumoniae*, nontypeable *Haemophilus influenzae*, and *Moraxella catarrhalis*. Many clinicians consider bacterial pneumonia, particularly *S. pneumoniae*, to be the likely cause of lower respiratory infection if the clinical history is characterized by acute onset of symptoms such as cough and high fever. In regard to the atypical pathogens, there is an age-related decline in the incidence of viral pneumonia accompanied by an increased incidence of these infections as children approach adolescence.

PRESENTATION

Recent reviews have suggested that the presence of an increased respiratory rate may be the best method to distinguish lower respiratory tract infection from the more common upper respiratory tract infections. The World Health Organization has issued guidelines for the clinical diagnosis of pneumonia in developing countries; the guidelines state that tachypnea and intercostal retractions are the best indications of lower respiratory tract disease.

DIAGNOSIS

Basic Diagnostic Approach

The proportion of children with pneumonia who are diagnosed with a specific etiology is low. Unlike adults, children usually do not produce adequate sputum specimens for Gram stain and culture. Blood cultures have a yield of less than 10% in patients with bacterial pneumonia. "Lung puncture" studies that are conducted in developing countries are obviously not met with enthusiasm in general pediatric practices. Prospective studies that have employed sensitive antibody tests and polymerase chain reaction techniques have suggested that in up to 20% of pediatric community-acquired pneumonias, the infection is "mixed" (i.e., both *S. pneumoniae* and *M. pneumoniae* or *C. pneumoniae*); in these cases, the primary pathogen is not clear. Authors of these studies have also suggested that mixed infection with bacteria and respiratory viruses is likely to be common as well.

Laboratory Findings

Many studies have looked at causes of pediatric pneumonia as it relates to certain readily available laboratory measurements. Many clinicians consider *S. pneumoniae* to be the likely cause of the lower respiratory infection if the picture is characterized by acute onset of high fever, lobar pneumonia on chest radiograph, leukocytosis, and a rapid response to β-lactam antibiotics. Numerous studies have found that chest radiographs do not readily distinguish between bacterial, atypical bacterial, and viral pneumonia. A variety of laboratory tests have been used in the attempt to distinguish bacterial from viral pneumonia, including the C-reactive protein and absolute neutrophil counts. One problem in using "screening" tests is that specific cutoff levels have often not been established. A recent study done in Europe found that although white blood cell count and C-reactive proteins were statistically higher in patients with pneumococcal infections, other clinical and laboratory and radiographic studies were of little value.

Given the clinical, epidemiologic, and laboratory difficulties in pinpointing the cause of pediatric pneumonia, an additional approach is to divide patients by age.

NEONATAL PNEUMONIA

Etiology

The primary bacterial pathogen in neonatal pneumonia is group B streptococci, although *Escherichia coli* and *Listeria monocytogenes* have also been reported. The mechanism is similar to that in neonatal sepsis, where colonization from the mother results in neonatal colonization and breakthrough infection.

Chlamydia trachomatis is the most common sexually transmitted infection in the United States. The organism may reside in the genital tract of pregnant women and be transmitted in about 60% of cases to infants at the time of delivery. About one half of infants who acquire the organism develop conjunctivitis, and 20% eventually develop lower respiratory disease.

Presentation

Pneumonia caused by bacteria such as group B streptococcus typically occurs in the first weeks of life, presenting with fever, increased work of breathing, and hypoxia. *C. trachomatis* infection usually occurs between 2 and 19 weeks after birth. The infants are afebrile, have increased respiratory rate, and cough. Children with chlamydial pneumonia often have hyperinflation, and bilateral infiltrates on chest x-ray, eosinophilia, and elevated serum immunoglobulin levels.

Diagnosis

Cultures of the blood, urine, and even cerebrospinal fluid are often obtained and intravenous antibiotic started. *C. trachomatis* can be diagnosed by culture or direct fluorescent antibody staining of nasopharyngeal secretions.

Management

The management of the febrile tachypneic neonate suspected of having pneumonia is similar to that of neonatal fever. Empiric intravenous antibiotics are started until culture results are final. Empiric treatment usually consists of ampicillin combined with gentamicin or a third-generation cephalosporin. Treatment of *C. trachomatis* is with oral erythromycin, 50 mg/kg per day in four divided doses for 2 weeks. In the past, erythromycin was given to neonates exposed to *C. trachomatis* at the time of delivery. Recently, there has been an association reported between oral erythromycin and the subsequent development of hypertrophic pyloric stenosis in infants younger than 6 weeks of age. The current recommendation is to treat with oral erythromycin, 50 mg/kg per day in four divided doses for 14 days all infants with chlamydial conjunctivitis and pneumonia. Patients who are exposed at the time of delivery are not presumptively treated, but rather monitored closely for the development of disease. Routine screening of all pregnant women for sexually transmitted disease is helpful in reducing disease by *C. trachomatis.*

PNEUMONIA IN THE FIRST 3 MONTHS OF LIFE

Respiratory Syncytial Virus

The peak incidence of this viral pathogen is in the first 6 months of life. Respiratory syncytial virus (RSV) typically occurs annually during the winter months. The spectrum of disease includes significant bronchiolitis and pneumonia in infants and younger children to a mild upper respiratory infection in older children. Patients with underlying conditions such as bronchopulmonary dysplasia, congenital heart disease, or underlying immunodeficiency are at risk for a more severe course.

RSV is diagnosed rapidly using a direct fluorescent antibody on nasal secretions. An aerosolized antibiotic agent, ribavirin, has been used in the treatment of RSV disease in infants. The use of ribavirin remains the subject of continuing debate. Citing new evidence, the American Academy of Pediatrics changed its recommendation in the 1990s regarding the use of ribavirin and now has a less stringent "may be considered" recommendation for its use in RSV infections in children with underlying conditions such as immunodeficiency, congenital heart disease, or chronic lung disease. Children with less serious disease need only supportive treatment.

Parainfluenza Virus

Parainfluenza viruses are very similar to the disease caused by RSV infection, but usually seen in the summer months. These viruses frequently cause croup but may also cause lower respiratory disease.

Streptococcus pneumoniae Infection

S. pneumoniae is the most common cause of bacterial pneumonia in this age group. This pathogen is often associated with sudden onset of cough and high fever. Leukocytosis is often present. Radiographs can show a discrete lobar pneumonia or round infiltrate; this in the proper clinical context suggests the diagnosis.

Pertussis

Pertussis is seen in this age group owing to absent or incomplete immunizations. Patients can present first with coryza (catarrhal stage) and then progress to cough (paroxysmal stage). Infants may also present with apnea or seizures. Lymphocytosis is frequently seen. The organism is difficult to culture and often not present during the paroxysmal phase of the illness. The diagnosis is made by direct immunofluorescence or polymerase chain reaction of nasal secretions. Treatment is with erythromycin. Newer macrolide antibiotics can be used, although there is less experience with these drugs.

PNEUMONIA IN CHILDREN 4 MONTHS TO 5 YEARS OF AGE

Viral pathogens again predominate in this age group, with RSV, parainfluenza, influenza, and adenovirus being common pathogens. The primary bacteria causing pneumonia in infants and children remains *S. pneumoniae*. Some studies also report *M. catarrhalis*, and nontypeable *H. influenzae* as pathogens.

PNEUMONIA IN CHILDREN 5 YEARS OF AGE AND OLDER

In this age group, the atypical pneumonias begin to be important agents. *S. pneumoniae* also remains a major cause of lower respiratory infection in this age group.

M. pneumoniae may begin with an upper respiratory infection that gradually progresses to pneumonia. Cough is frequently a persistent symptom. Although *M. pneumoniae* is classically a respiratory infection, additional extrapulmonary manifestations are seen and include encephalitis, hemolytic anemia, and Stevens-Johnson syndrome. Serology is usually the method for diagnosis.

C. pneumoniae was formerly termed TWAR strain. A sore throat or history of hoarseness usually precedes the onset of lower respiratory infection and can be a clue to diagnosis. Illness may run a protracted course lasting several weeks. The diagnosis of the *C. pneumoniae* is made by serology.

L. pneumophila is another pathogen associated with the atypical pneumonia group. Outbreaks are often associated with exposure to water contaminated by the organism because it tends to grow in water systems and air conditioning. *Legionella* species are difficult to culture; it needs special buffer charcoal yeast extract (BCYE agar) to support growth in the laboratory. Laboratories should always be informed if *Legionella* species infection is suspected. Patients who are hospitalized with severe disease can undergo bronchoscopy for culture of bronchial alveolar fluids. In addition to serology, direct fluorescent antibodies of bronchial alveolar washings and urinary antigen testing are also available for diagnosis.

The atypical pathogens are treated differently from the other bacterial pneumonias, relying on the use of either tetracycline or macrolide antibiotics. Efforts have been made to devise a clinical scoring system that will identify the atypical pathogen in the moderate to severely ill patient with community-based pneumonia. Some studies have found high temperature and previous unsuccessful therapy with β-lactam antibiotics as being predictive of atypical pneumonia. Other studies have not been able to differentiate reliably between the two groups of lower respiratory infection. If there is a concern regarding etiology in a moderately to severely ill patient, specific testing by serology, urinary antigen, or bronchoscopy is advised.

TREATMENT OF COMMUNITY-ACQUIRED PNEUMONIA

The evaluation and empiric treatment of pediatric community-acquired pneumonia has been the subject of numerous reviews. Investigators agree that clinical evaluation forms the foundation for practice. If a child is nontoxic and has obvious signs of a viral infection (such as rhinorrhea and nonexudative pharyngitis), no antibiotics are required, and close follow-up is advocated.

In a young child who is suspected of having a bacterial illness (i.e., persistent fever), but who has good hydration status and adequate oxygenation, empiric antibiotics are appropriate. Treatment with oral antibiotics is usually directed against *S. pneumoniae* because this is the most common cause of bacterial pneumonia in children. During the past decade, alterations in penicillin-binding proteins have led to increasing resistance of the pneumococci to both penicillin and the cephalosporins. Increasing minimal inhibitory concentration (MIC) to β-lactam antibiotics has resulted in new recommendations for the treatment of *S. pneumoniae* meningitis. Lower respiratory infection differs from meningitis in that there is no blood–brain barrier and therefore no reduction of antibiotic concentration in the infected space. The MIC of *S. pneumoniae* can thus be interpreted differently in pneumonia than in meningitis. In regard to penicillin, *S. pneumoniae* is reported as susceptible (MIC ≤ .06 μg/mL), intermediate (0.12 to 1.0 μg/mL), and resistant (>2.0 μg/mL). Unlike the therapy of meningitis, lower respiratory infections caused by intermediate strains will usually respond to penicillin and other β-lactam antibiotics. Pneumonia caused by resistant strains may not be effectively treated by penicillin or even third-generation cephalosporins. In these cases, alternate agents such as vancomycin or fluoroquinolones may be required. An *S. pneumoniae* isolate with an MIC to cefotaxime of 2.0 μg/mL or less can be treated with a third-generation cephalosporin.

In children older than 5 years of age, consideration of *M. pneumoniae* is required. Empiric treatment with a macrolide has been proposed for this age group. Pneumococcal resistance to macrolide antibiotics is also increasing, with two separate mechanisms of resistance identified. *S. pneumoniae* resistance to macrolide may be secondary to alterations in drug-binding sites or the development of active drug efflux. Although the overall *in vitro* resistance rate of *S. pneumoniae* to macrolides approaches 30%, it is not clear whether this correlates with clinical failure. It has been suggested that the clinical effect of *in vitro* macrolide resistance may depend on the precise mechanism of resistance present in the infecting organism or the presence of concurrent bacteremic disease. Macrolide therapy for presumed *S. pneumoniae* lower respiratory disease is reasonable in a stable outpatient population; children who are toxic, bacteremic, or fail to improve after macrolide monotherapy may warrant combination therapy with β-lactam antibiotics.

TABLE 13.1. *Empiric Treatment for Community Acquired Pneumonia*

1. Associated with signs of viral illness (coryza, pharyngitis)	No treatment
2. Continued symptoms, moderate toxicity but not needing hospitalization	
a. 4 mo–5 yrs	a. High-dose amoxicillin (80–90 mg/kg/d in divided doses) b. Augmentin (amoxicillin-clavulanate) c. Oral second- or third-generation cephalosporin
b. >5 yrs Needs consideration of *Mycoplasma pneumonia*	a. Clarithromycin (15 mg/kg/d in 2 divided doses) or azithromycin (10 mg/kg, then 5 mg/kg for 4 d) b. If no improvement, consider treatment as per 2a
3. Children requiring hospitalization	a. Clindamycin or Unasyn (ampicillin-sulbactam) or a third-generation cephalosporin b. Mycoplasma treatment with macrolide antibiotics c. If child toxic or with life-threatening disease, consider vancomycin and third-generation cephalosporin in addition to macrolide antibiotic

In children who are toxic appearing, hypoxic, or require intravenous hydration, treatment is directed toward both atypical pathogens and bacteria causing severe pyogenic pneumonia, including *Streptococcus pyogenes*, *S. pneumoniae*, and *Staphylococcus aureus*. In treating pneumonia in a toxic-appearing child, the clinician must remember the increasing incidence of resistance in both community *S. aureus* (MRSA) and *S. pneumoniae* (MIC to penicillin $\geq$ 2.0 µg/mL). Vancomycin and a third-generation cephalosporin are reasonable initial therapy in the case of a potentially life-threatening lower respiratory infection. For children who are not in critical condition, a third-generation cephalosporin, clindamycin, or ampicillin-sulbactam (Unasyn) is an acceptable choice. A macrolide antibiotic will also be needed for treatment of the atypical pneumonia pathogens (Table 13.1).

PARAPNEUMONIC EFFUSIONS AND EMPYEMA

Bacterial pneumonia can have a variety of complications. A parapneumonic effusion refers to pleural fluid that accumulates in association with bacterial pneumonia. A certain percentage of these effusions will undergo a secondary process in which the fluid becomes purulent and, if untreated, will actually form a pleural peel that adheres to the surface of the lung. At this stage, the parapneumonic effusion is typically referred to as an *empyema*.

Etiology

The three major bacteria responsible for parapneumonic effusion and empyema are *S. aureus, S. pneumoniae,* and *S. pyogenes* (group A streptococci). The rate of empyema varies with each particular bacterium; group A streptococcus pneumonia progresses to empyema in up to 40% of patients, whereas less than 5% of patients with pneumococcal pneumonia develop an empyema.

Clinical and Radiographic Features

Patients with parapneumonic effusions or empyema often continue to have spiking temperatures despite appropriate antibiotics. Chest x-ray is usually the initial step in evaluating this condition. If there is extensive effusion, the chest radiograph may appear as a "whiteout," the entire side of the lung becomes opaque. In these cases, computed tomography of the chest is excellent in distinguishing pleural from parenchymal disease. Computed tomography can also detect the presence of large loculations (Figs. 13.1 and 13.2).

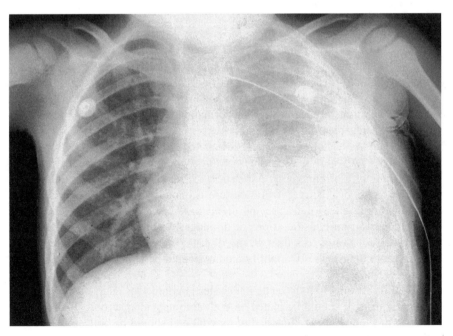

FIG. 13.1. Plain radiograph showing complete opacification of left lung consistent with empyema.

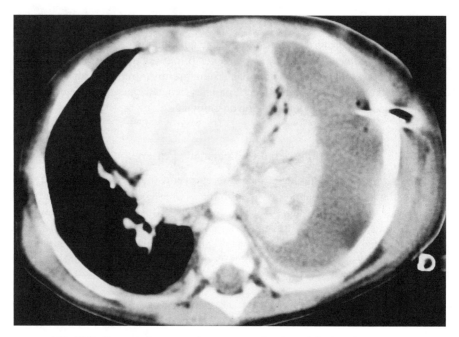

FIG. 13.2. Computed tomography scan revealing large left pleural empyema.

Diagnosis

Once a pleural effusion has been identified, analysis of the pleural effusion is necessary. A common mistake is to delay evaluation and drainage of pleural effusion; this can ultimately lead to further formation of loculations and greater difficulty in ultimately clearing the infection.

Because treatment of empyema requires not only antibiotic therapy but also surgical drainage, there is great interest in the pleural fluid parameters that define the diagnosis of empyema. Aspiration of frankly purulent material, a positive Gram stain, or positive pleural culture is enough to make a definitive diagnosis. In the absence of frankly purulent material, there are changes that, of themselves, warrant consideration for drainage. A pleural fluid pH of less than 7.2, a glucose level of less than 40 mg/dL, and a lactate dehydrogenase (LDH) level of more than 1,000 IU identify a complicated parapneumonic effusion that requires drainage.

Pleural fluid should be obtained under sterile conditions and sent for a variety of specific tests. It should be plated on both aerobic and anaerobic media. Determination of the pH of the pleural fluid is vital and should be collected anaerobically and transported on ice to the laboratory. Cell count and chemical analysis are also important.

TABLE 13.2. *Diagnosis and Management of Empyema*

1. Child with fever, hypoxia, decreased breath sounds
2. Chest radiograph—pleural effusion or "white out"
3. Computed tomography scan of chest (if needed) to distinguish pleural effusion from parenchymal disease
4. Diagnostic thoracentesis or (if high suspicion of empyema) immediate chest tube placement
5. Pleural fluid evaluation (chest tube indicated if any of the following present)
   a. Grossly purulent fluid
   b. pH < 7.2
   c. Lactate dehydrogenase > 1,000 IU
   d. Glucose < 40 mg/dL
   e. Positive Gram stain or culture
6. If patient is persistently febrile despite chest tube, consider video-assisted thoracic surgery (VATS) or open thoracotomy for decortication

Management

Treatment of Empyema

In patients in whom an empyema is diagnosed, either by pH, LDH, glucose, Gram stain, or the documentation of gross pus within the pleural space, at the very **least** a chest tube is required for continued drainage. If the initial suspicion for empyema is high, initial diagnostic thoracentesis may be replaced by immediate placement of a chest tube. In most cases, chest tubes can be removed when the amount of pleural fluid draining from the tube has decreased and the effusion has resolved on plain x-ray. There will be a percentage of patients who do not clear the empyema with chest tube drainage alone. These patients are candidates for further surgical intervention. Patients who require surgical intervention typically have persistent fever, toxicity, and minimal chest tube drainage. These patients often have developed loculations that are not amenable to drainage by chest tube.

In the past, thoracotomy and decortication was done. In this procedure, the chest is opened, pleura removed, and purulent material evacuated from the pleural space. Video-assisted thoracic surgery (VATS) is being increasingly used; this procedure has the advantage of a smaller surgical incision and fewer complications. A greater number of pediatric surgeons are advocating earlier use of VATS, even before placement of a chest tube, for the initial treatment of pediatric empyema. As experience with VATS increases, it may be prudent to involve an experienced pediatric surgeon as soon as a pleural empyema is diagnosed (Table 13.2).

SELECTED READINGS

Campbell JD, Nataro JP. Pleural empyema. *Pediatr Infect Dis J* 1999;18(8):725–726.
Gaston B. Pneumonia. *Pediatr Rev* 2002;23(4):132–140.
McCracken GH. Diagnosis and management of pneumonia in children. *Pediatr Infect Dis* J 2000;(9): 924–928.
Rodriguez JA, Hill CB, Loe WA, et al. Video-assisted thoracoscopic surgery for children with stage II empyema. *Am Surg* 2000;66(6):569–572.

14

Salmonella Gastroenteritis

EPIDEMIOLOGY

Salmonella has more than 2,000 serotypes. Although one can attempt to memorize all of them, a more practical method is to divide salmonella into two basic categories: invasive (enteric fever) and noninvasive (nontyphoidal). These categories are different in transmission, presentation, and management.

ENTERIC FEVER

Invasive salmonella refers mainly to *Salmonella typhi*, although other salmonella serotypes can cause invasive disease. *S. typhi* is found only in humans and is spread person to person. These serotypes have certain antigens that allow them to become invasive from the gastrointestinal tract, causing a prolonged bacteremic illness. This bacteremic illness is referred to as **enteric fever** or **typhoid fever**.

Presentation

Infected patients often have fever, leukopenia, hepatosplenomegaly, and abdominal distention. Diarrhea can occur, but because the bacteria is invasive and does not reside long in the gastrointestinal tract, constipation can also be noted. "Rose spots" represent embolic salmonella to the skin and are rare in children. A major issue in typhoid fever is early consideration. Typhoid fever should be considered in any child with a fever and recent travel to an endemic area. This is particularly true if the child has hepatosplenomegaly, leukopenia, and negative malarial smears. Typhoid fever is frequently misdiagnosed as malaria because the endemic regions are similar and both may present with high, spiking fever.

Diagnosis

Diagnosis of enteric fever rests on isolation of the organism from blood culture. Blood cultures are positive in a large percentage of patients. Stool cultures can also be positive and may be diagnostic in the correct clinical setting. Febrile agglutinins

(Widal's test) have previously been used, with elevation of O and H titers greater than 1:160 being diagnostic. Currently, these tests are not recommended owing to high rates of false-positive and false-negative results.

Treatment of Invasive Disease

Patients with invasive salmonella disease should always be treated. An increasing percentage of isolates are resistant to ampicillin and trimethoprim-sulfamethoxazole (Bactrim), traditionally the front-line antibiotics for treatment of this organism. Treatment is usually initiated with a third-generation cephalosporin such as cefotaxime or ceftriaxone. Second-generation cephalosporins and gentamicin are not considered efficacious, although *in vitro* assays may show sensitivity. Fluoroquinolones such as ciprofloxacin are frequently used for treatment of invasive salmonella disease, particularly in developing countries.

Chronic Infection

About 3% of patients infected with typhoid fever develop chronic infection. This is defined as excretions in the stool for longer than 1 year. Chronic infection serves as a nidus for subsequent infection in others and can be extremely difficult to eradicate. Some children respond to high-dose intravenous ampicillin or oral amoxicillin. In adult chronic carriers, ciprofloxacin is used, often with adjunctive cholecystectomy.

Invasive Salmonella: *Salmonella typhi*

- Causes enteric fever
- Person-to-person spread
- Chronic carrier state
- Fever, leukopenia, abdominal pain, hepatomegaly
- Treatment always indicated

NONTYPHOIDAL SALMONELLA

Etiology

Nontyphoidal salmonella refers to noninvasive disease. The most common illness caused by nontyphoidal salmonella is gastroenteritis. These organisms are found principally in food and animals. A percentage of food products, including eggs and chicken, are contaminated with salmonella strains. Pets, including turtles and iguanas, are also a well-described reservoir for nontyphoidal salmonella.

Once infected, prolonged excretion can occur, particularly in children. Almost half of children younger than 5 years of age continue to shed salmonella months after initial infection. It has been found that antibiotic therapy can actually prolong this excretion. It has been speculated that antibiotics suppress the protective effects of indigenous intestinal bacteria, which results in the continued survival and excretion of the salmonella bacteria. Unlike with *S. typhi*, chronic infection does not occur. Routine administration of antibiotics for salmonella gastroenteritis is not recommended because they are not thought to reduce clinical illness and can prolong excretion of the organism.

Presentation

The most common manifestation of nontyphoidal salmonella infection is gastroenteritis. Although nontyphoid salmonella infections are usually confined to the gastrointestinal tract, there are variations in the clinical course. In young children, nontyphoid salmonella can behave very much like invasive salmonella strains. A percentage of young children with salmonella gastroenteritis have concurrent bacteremia. The reported incidence of bacteremia in children with nontyphoid salmonella gastroenteritis has been reported to be from 5% to 45%. This bacteremia can potentially result in severe morbidity and mortality from resultant osteomyelitis, sepsis, and meningitis. In general, a higher incidence of bacteremia is found in children younger than 1 year of age.

Diagnosis

Given the incidence of concurrent bacteremia, an index of suspicion for salmonella gastroenteritis and bacteremia should be had in evaluating a young child, particularly in the first year of life. Numerous studies have addressed the clinical predictors that can be used for acute bacterial diarrhea in young children. The best predictive variable for a stool culture positive for bacterial pathogen is the presence of polymorphonuclear cells in the stools. Three symptoms useful in distinguishing bacterial from viral gastroenteritis are an abrupt onset of diarrhea, more than four stools per day, and no vomiting before the onset of diarrhea. A young child with high fever and gastroenteritis in whom bacterial disease is possible should have a stool and blood culture obtained.

Management

Bacteremic illness should always be treated, usually for 10 to 14 days. In febrile children in the first year of life with proven salmonella gastroenteritis, even without bacteremia, treatment should be considered. This is particularly true in children with underlying conditions such as human immunodeficiency virus (HIV) infection or sickle cell anemia and in those receiving immunosuppressive therapy.

Noninvasive Salmonella

- Food-borne illness
- No chronic carrier state
- Usually causes self-limited gastroenteritis
- Antibiotics usually not indicated

SELECTED READINGS

Katz BZ, Shapiro ED. Predictors of persistently positive blood cultures in children with "occult" salmonella bacteremia. *Pediatr Infect Dis* 1986;5(6):713–714.

Stormon MO, McIntyre PB, Morris J, et al. Typhoid fever in children: diagnostic and therapeutic difficulties. *Pediatr Infect Dis J* 1997;16(7):713–714.

Zaidi E, Bachur R, Harper M. Non-typhi Salmonella bacteremia in children. *Pediatr Infect Dis J* 1999;18(12):1073–1077.

15

Catheter Infection

The use of long-term indwelling catheters has revolutionized medical care. Chemotherapy, as well as prolonged antimicrobial treatment and parenteral nutrition, can be given without repeated replacement of peripheral catheters. However, catheter infection remains a major cause of morbidity in these patients.

EPIDEMIOLOGY

The most common mechanism of catheter infection is the colonization by bacteria at the insertion site with subsequent migration to the catheter tip. A less frequent cause of catheter infection is the hematogenous seeding of the catheter from a bacteremia originating at a separate site.

PRESENTATION

Consideration of catheter infection should be made in all patients with indwelling catheters presenting with fever. This is particularly true in patients who have signs of inflammation around the catheter itself. The evaluation of a febrile patient who has an indwelling catheter should always include the following:

1. **Vital signs.** Decreased peripheral perfusion and hypotension may be signs of progressive sepsis and should always be part of the evaluation.
2. **Timing of catheter placement.** Patients who have had catheter placement within the past 2 to 3 weeks are at a higher risk for infection with *Staphylococcus aureus*.
3. **History of previous catheter infection.** A patient recently completing antibiotic therapy, especially if the treatment did not include catheter removal, may be presenting with a relapsed infection with the **same** organism.
4. **Any other explanations for fever, including signs of upper or lower respiratory infection.**

DIAGNOSIS OF CATHETER INFECTIONS

The hallmark of the diagnosis of catheter infection is a positive blood culture from the catheter. One of the challenges is that the blood culture may be positive in a patient with a catheter who has a catheter infection **or** has sepsis originating at a separate site. Furthermore, a bacteremia originating at another site may ultimately seed and infect that catheter.

Several methods have been proposed for the diagnosis of catheter infection:

1. **Culture of the catheter tip** is a common method used for the diagnosis of catheter infection. In the semiquantitative method, the catheter segment is rolled across the agar plate, and colony-forming units are counted after 24 hours of incubation. The quantitative method of catheter culture is done by flushing or vortexing the catheter segment with broth, followed by serial dilution or plating on an agar plate. A colony count of at least 15 colony-forming units by semiquantitative method or at least 100 colony-forming units from the quantitative method is indicative of catheter infection. An obvious disadvantage of this method is that the catheter has to be removed before the diagnosis of infection can be confirmed.

2. **Paired quantitative blood cultures.** Patients in whom catheter infection is considered should always have two sets of blood cultures obtained: a blood culture from the catheter in question and a peripheral blood culture. A blood culture from an infected catheter should have 5 to 10 times more colony-forming units per cc than the peripheral blood culture. The use of paired quantitative blood cultures offers the advantage of evaluating for catheter infection without removal of the catheter.

3. **Time to positivity**. New technology in the processing of blood cultures allows for continuous monitoring, allowing for a time to positivity to be documented. It has been reported that there is a difference between the time to positivity between blood cultures from peripheral veins and blood cultures obtained from infected catheters. This time difference is related to the size in the inoculum of bacteria between a blood culture obtained through an infected catheter and that from a peripheral site. A time difference of greater than 2 hours is highly sensitive for the diagnosis of catheter-related infection. A limitation to this methodology is that an ability to monitor the automated blood culture system must be available.

4. **Persistent positive cultures**. This is often one of the most practical ways of proving a catheter infection. Repeated positive cultures through the catheter despite the administration of appropriate antibiotics strongly suggests a source of infection, the source usually being the catheter itself. After 48 to 72 hours of appropriate antibiotic treatment, continued positive blood cultures through the catheter suggest the diagnosis of catheter infection.

A summary of the diagnostic methods for catheter infection is provided in Table 15.1.

TABLE 15.1. *Diagnosis of Catheter Infections*

	Diagnosis
1. Culture of removed catheter	
a. Semiquantitative method	≥15 CFU
b. Quantitative method	≥100 CFU
2. Paired blood cultures	
Simultaneous blood cultures done from catheter and peripheral vein	5–10 times difference in colony count between central and peripheral cultures
3. Time to "positivity"	≥2 h difference in time to positivity of culture from catheter to that of peripheral culture
4. Continual bacteremia	Persistent bacteremia on appropriate antimicrobial therapy suggests catheter injection

MANAGEMENT

Empiric Antibiotic Therapy

Depending on the clinical status of the patient, empiric therapy should be broad. Many clinicians, when faced with a potential catheter infection, include vancomycin (as coverage for coagulase-negative staphylococcus, *S. aureus,* methicillin-resistant *S. aureus,* and enterococcus). Some physicians who wish to limit the empiric use of vancomycin begin with semisynthetic penicillin such as nafcillin and resort to vancomycin only when a pathogen requiring vancomycin is documented. Because of the rapid mortality caused by gram-negative organisms, aggressive gram-negative coverage is usually begun. This often consists of a third-generation cephalosporin combined with an aminoglycoside. In patients who are severely ill, with decreased peripheral profusion and hypotension, empiric antifungal treatment may be started. The initial empiric therapy can always be reduced after culture results are available.

Treatment of Catheter Infections

There are two options for the treatment of catheter infections:

1. Antibiotic therapy alone
2. Catheter removal with antibiotic therapy

Organisms that infect catheters often produce a biofilm that causes the organism to adhere to the catheter. It has been shown that antibiotic concentration must be 100 to 1,000 times greater to kill bacteria residing within a biofilm. This explains the difficulty in treating infected catheters with antibiotic therapy alone.

Guidelines have recently been published by the Infectious Disease Society of America. This important document states that randomized trials regarding treatment of infected catheters are lacking; definitive recommendations therefore are often not available. Recommendations are based on a consensus from a panel of experts, taking into account a large amount of historical experience with catheter infections. These guidelines are grouped according to the pathogens causing the catheter infection.

It is important to remember that a clinical or microbiological relapse following completion of antibiotics with the same pathogen in a patient in whom the catheter was retained, warrants immediate consideration for catheter removal, regardless of the pathogen.

SPECIFIC PATHOGENS OF CATHETER INFECTION

Coagulase-negative *Staphylococcus*

Coagulase-negative staphylococci are the most common cause of catheter infection. These bacteria may have lower virulence than other pathogens, and one can consider treatment with antibiotic therapy alone. The treatment is with oxacillin or nafcillin for methicillin-sensitive isolates and with vancomycin for organisms that are methicillin resistant. Some investigators believe that infection with coagulase-negative staphylococcus represents an infection with a heterogenous population of organisms; that is, the organisms involved in the infection may be both oxacillin sensitive and resistant. Thus, some clinicians use vancomycin for any coagulase-negative staphylococcus infection thought to require treatment. Treatment is for 10 to 14 days in patients in whom the catheter is retained.

Staphylococcus aureus

S. aureus is a pathogen of higher virulence, often associated with secondary seeding (i.e., endocarditis and osteomyelitis). Many clinicians believe the treatment of an *S. aureus* catheter infection with antibiotics alone is difficult and often results in continued bacteremia and increased risk for infection of secondary sites. The most current recommendation includes removal of the catheter and antibiotic therapy for 14 days.

The diagnosis of endocarditis in patients with *S. aureus* bacteremia remains controversial. In adults, transesophageal echocardiography (TEE) is routinely used to assess for vegetations. In patients who have had a prolonged course of bacteremia or have abnormalities on TEE, treatment with antibiotics is often given for 4 to 6 weeks.

In pediatrics, the use of TEE is limited, making the diagnosis of *S. aureus* endocarditis more difficult. Some clinicians, when faced with persistent bacteremia preceding or following catheter removal, make a presumptive diagnosis of endocarditis and consider a prolonged course of antibiotic therapy.

Gram-negative Bacilli

The gram-negative bacilli are increasingly causing catheter-related infections. No controlled studies have addressed definitively whether catheters infected by gram-negative bacilli must be removed. In some settings in which the patient is hemodynamically stable, attempts with medical therapy alone can be tried. In patients who present with a septic picture, hypotension, or system failure, immediate catheter removal should be considered. A recent study examining gram-negative catheter infection in neonates found that the bacteremia was successfully treated with medical management in only 45% of cases; successful therapy was most likely to occur when there was only a single day's duration of bacteremia. Infection was rarely resolved in infants who had more prolonged bacteremia and bacteremia-associated thrombocytopenia, unless the catheter was removed.

Candida Species

Candida species are another major cause of morbidity and mortality in patients with catheter infections. Once a fungal catheter infection is documented, removal of the catheter is necessary. Retention of the catheter will only result in persistent fungemia, which can cause significant morbidity and even mortality.

Although minimal inhibitory concentration (MIC) breakpoints are not available for amphotericin B, breakpoints for candidal species to the azole class (e.g., fluconazole, itraconazole) are available. The Infectious Disease Society of America has recently published recommendations regarding the treatment of a variety of *Candida* species with antifungal agents. Infections with *Candida albicans, Candida tropicalis,* and *Candida parapsilosis* can usually be treated with fluconazole. *Candida krusei* and *Candida glabrata* are generally considered resistant to fluconazole and may have reduced sensitivity to amphotericin B, requiring either increased dosing of amphotericin B or the use of caspofungin. *Candida lusitaniae* is considered to be potentially resistant to amphotericin B. Current guidelines recognize that resistance patterns may change over time; testing for azole resistance may need to be increasingly used, particularly if faced with clinical or microbiological failure.

Duration of therapy for fungemia is a common question. Adequate therapy is desired because of the high risk for secondary spread to bone, kidneys, or cerebrospinal fluid. In the past, all fungemia was treated with a 6-week course of antifungal agents. Recently, efforts to determine which patients may be candidates for a shorter course of antifungal therapy have been made. Early catheter removal is essential. A vigorous search for secondary sites of infection by urine culture, urinalysis, funduscopic examination, and renal ultrasound are often recommended. If repeat blood cultures following catheter removal are negative and there is no evidence of a secondary infected site, many clinicians will administer 2 weeks of additional therapy following first negative culture. Secondary sites of infection need prolonged therapy (Table 15.2).

Routine Changes of Central Venous Catheters

Recently, several studies have examined the prevention of catheter-related bloodstream infections in the intensive care setting with scheduled replacement of these

TABLE 15.2. *Management of Catheter Infections by Specific Pathogens*

Pathogen	Treatment
Coagulase-negative staphylococcus	1. Catheter retention: antibiotics for 10–14 d 2. Catheter removed: antibiotic treatment for 5–7 d
Staphylococcus aureus	1. Catheter removal with antibiotic treatment for 14 d 2. If evidence of secondary disease (positive echocardiogram, persistent bacteria), treat with antibiotics for 4–6 wks
Gram-negative bacilli	1. Catheter removal and antibiotic treatment for 10–14 d
Candida species	1. Catheter removal and antifungal therapy for a minimum of 14 d 2. Fluconazole-resistant *Candida* species (*C. krusei, C. glabrata*) may require amphotericin B or caspofungin therapy 3. *Candida lusitaniae* usually amphotericin B resistant

catheters over guide wires. These studies have not shown a decrease in infection; there was actually an increased risk for mechanical complication when the catheters were replaced. The most current recommendation is that routine scheduling and changing of catheters does not prevent catheter-related bloodstream infections.

SELECTED READINGS

Benjamin, DK, Miller W, Garges H, et al. Bacteremia, central catheters, and neonates: when to pull the line. *Pediatrics* 2001;107(6):1272–1276.

Donowitz LG, Hendley JO. Short course amphotericin B therapy for candidemia in pediatric patients. *Pediatrics* 1995;95(6):888–891.

Gaur AH, Flynn PM, Giannini MA, et al. Difference in time to detection: a simple method to differentiate catheter-related from non-catheter related blood steam infection in immunocompromised pediatric patients. *Clin Infect Dis* 2003;37(4):469–475.

Haimi-Cohen Y, Shafinoori S, Tucci V, et al. Use of incubation time to detect in BACTEC 9240 to distinguish coagulase-negative staphylococcal contamination from infection in pediatric blood cultures. *Pediatr Infect Dis J* 2003;22:968–973.

Mermel LA, Farr BM, Sheretz RJ, et al. Guidelines for the management of intravascular catheter-related infections. *Clin Infect Dis* 2001;32(9):1249–1272.

Nazemi KJ, Buescher ES, Kelly RE, et al. Central venous catheter removal versus in situ treatment in neonates with Enterobacteriaceae bacteremia. *Pediatrics* 2003;111(3):E269–274.

16

Infection in Unusual Spaces

Certain pediatric infections are noteworthy for their presence in unusual body spaces. These may be rarely seen but when present require rapid diagnosis and therapy. This chapter provides a discussion of such infections, including necrotizing fasciitis, omphalitis, endophthalmitis, peritonitis secondary to ruptured appendicitis, and retropharyngeal abscess.

NECROTIZING FASCIITIS

Necrotizing fasciitis is an infection involving the subcutaneous tissues and deep fascia. It can affect any portion of the body, although the lower extremities are the most commonly involved. First described by Hippocrates in the 5th century, this condition has been reported under a variety of names, including "hospital gangrene" and "malignant ulcer." The term necrotizing fasciitis was first used in the 1950s and accurately describes the location of infection.

Etiology

The infection begins with the introduction of the pathogen into the subcutaneous tissues. Many mechanisms of this introduction have been reported, including insect bites, minor trauma, preceding varicella infection, and surgical incisions. Hematogenous spread has also been reported as a means of inoculation. A variety of toxins, cytokines, and inflammatory mediators are thought to be involved in the progression of the infection.

Necrotizing fasciitis has been divided into distinct groups based on causative organism. Type 1 refers to a polymicrobial infection usually caused by non–group A streptococcus and other aerobic and anaerobic bacteria. Type II necrotizing fasciitis usually is caused by group A streptococcus alone or with staphylococcus. The etiologic agents of necrotizing fasciitis cannot be determined from clinical presentation alone. During the past decade, the most common cause of necrotizing fasciitis has remained group A streptococcus following varicella infection. It is thought that the group A streptococcus is inoculated directly into the skin when the child scratches the varicella lesions.

Presentation

A major challenge for the pediatrician is to separate necrotizing fasciitis from a routine cellulitis. Clinical examination is the mainstay of diagnosis. A major clue on physical examination involves severe pain, often out of proportion to the physical findings. As the infection progresses, one finds worsening erythema and edema. Later, the skin may develop blisters, and bullae may form (Fig. 16.1). The formation of bullae is thought to be an important diagnostic finding that should always raise the suspicion for necrotizing fasciitis. Later in the progression of the disease, the bullae become hemorrhagic and are often accompanied by crepitus.

Diagnosis

Several tests have been used in an attempt to document the progression of cellulitis to necrotizing fasciitis. The presence of leukocytosis and acidosis has been used to identify patients with progressive disease. The appearance of gas on plain radiograph is an inconsistent finding and is seen in less than 20% of cases. Magnetic resonance imaging (MRI) has been reported to detect extension of the inflammatory process into the subcutaneous tissue. High signal intensity of the fascia in the T2-weighted images strongly suggests the diagnosis.

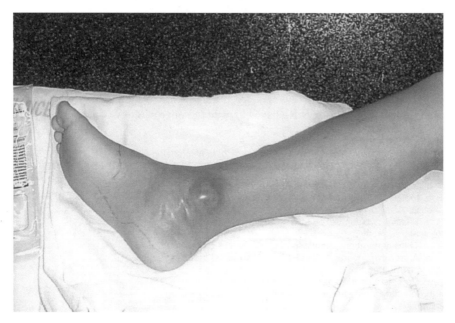

FIG. 16.1. Cellulitis, edema, and bullae formation in child with necrotizing fasciitis (see color plate).

The gold standard of diagnosis for necrotizing fasciitis is surgical biopsy; biopsies reveal acute inflammation of the dermis and fascia with accompanying thrombosis of blood vessels.

Management

The management of necrotizing fasciitis involves aggressive medical and surgical therapy. Optimal medical treatment includes a third-generation cephalosporin and anaerobic coverage, usually with clindamycin. Complete débridement of all devitalized tissue is required. A repeat second-look surgery after 24 hours is often needed to determine whether remaining devitalized tissue is present. Adjunctive therapies include hyperbaric oxygen and intravenous immunoglobulin, although definitive data of the efficacy of these measures is lacking (Table 16.1).

OMPHALITIS

Omphalitis, or infection of the umbilicus, remains a major cause of morbidity and mortality in developing countries. In a poorly understood process, omphalitis is thought to arise from bacterial colonization occurring at the time of delivery. This colonization becomes invasive and can proceed to **funisitis** (a term given to mild cellulitis or inflammation of the periumbilical skin) or to omphalitis, in which the umbilical stump and surrounding tissues are involved.

Etiology

Omphalitis has been traditionally caused by *Staphylococcus aureus* and *Streptococcus pyogenes* (group A streptococcus.) Modern cord care with triple-dye antimicrobial soap and alcohol has reduced the frequency of omphalitis in developed countries; however, it may also have changed the microbiology of omphalitis. Dur-

TABLE 16.1. *Management of Necrotizing Fasciitis*

Diagnosis
    a. Pain out of proportion to physical exam
    b. Induration, "woody" edema
    c. Leukocytosis, acidosis
    d. Fascial involvement on MRI
Medical treatment
    a. Third generation cephalosporin; cefotaxime 50 mg/kg IV q8
    b. Anaerobic coverage; Clindamycin 20-40 mg/kg/d divided q8
Surgical treatment
    a. Complete debridement of devitalized tissue
    b. "Second look" surgery may be needed
Adjunctive care
    a. Hyperbaric oxygen
    b. Intravenous immunoglobulin (400 mg/kg/dose)

ing the past 10 years, reports of omphalitis have emphasized the role of additional pathogens, particularly gram-negative and anaerobic bacteria.

Presentation

Neonates typically present with purulent discharge of the umbilical cord with rapidly progressing cellulitis of the abdominal wall.

Diagnosis

The diagnosis is based largely on the history and clinical examination. It is generally thought that any abdominal wall cellulitis surrounding the umbilical structures is consistent with the diagnosis of omphalitis.

Management

Due to the potential life-threatening complications of an umbilical cord infection, neonates presenting with any evidence of inflammation around the umbilical cord should be managed aggressively. This includes admission and treatment with broad-spectrum antibiotics, usually a third-generation cephalosporin and clindamycin. Surface cultures should be obtained, although it should be stressed that these may not represent the entire spectrum of bacteria involved in the deeper fascial planes. As in necrotizing fasciitis, surgical resection is a major part of therapy, and early involvement with experienced pediatric surgeons is mandatory.

Continued concern regarding omphalitis has led to an ongoing evaluation of optimal umbilical cord care. Some hospitals have abandoned triple-dye alcohol regimens for a regimen of dry cord care consisting of gentle cleaning with soap and water and allowing the area to air dry. A prospective study evaluating this approach in nearly 800 infants found a single case of omphalitis in the dry care group. In the dry care group, infants were more likely to be colonized with group B streptococcus, *S. aureus*, and gram-negative bacteria. Whether this colonization ultimately leads to an increase in invasive infection will need to be the subject of further studies (Table 16.2).

TABLE 16-2. *Management of Omphalitis*

Medical therapy
    a. Polymicrobial infection including S. aureus, group A streptococcus, anaerobes
    b. Surface cultures may not reflect all causative pathogens
    c. Cefotaxime – 100-200 mg/kg/day in 3 divided doses
    d. Clindamycin – 20-40 mg/kg/day in 3 divided doses
Surgical therapy
    a. Complete excision of affected tissue

ENDOPHTHALMITIS

Endophthalmitis refers to infection within the ocular structures. There are two mechanisms for this infection. In endogenous (hematogenous) endophthalmitis, bacteria are seeded within the eye following a bacteremic or septicemic illness. Exogenous endophthalmitis refers to infection within the eye following direct inoculation from a surgical procedure or traumatic event.

Etiology

Organisms that can seed the ocular structures following a bacteremic or septicemic illness include *Bacillus cereus, Candida* species, and *Neisseria meningitidis*. *B. cereus* infection is associated with the use of intravenous drugs. Organisms of exogenous disease include *Staphylococcus epidermidis, Streptococcus* species, and *S. aureus.*

Presentation

Patients have decreased vision and proptosis, often accompanied by periocular inflammation and edema. Visual acuity is usually markedly decreased. This process should be suspected in any bacteremic patient who, during the course of illness, develops ocular complaints. Exogenous endophthalmitis is particularly important in pediatrics because ocular trauma may not be immediately reported.

Diagnosis

The diagnosis of endophthalmitis should be done in conjunction with an experienced ophthalmologist. Ophthalmologic examination may reveal corneal haziness and a purulent exudate (hypopyon) in the anterior chamber of the eye. Typically, anterior chamber and vitreous aspiration should be performed in an effort to identify the responsible pathogen. The yield of Gram stain or culture approaches 60%.

Treatment

Therapy is difficult, given the low rate of positive cultures and the poor penetration of systemic antibiotics into the eye. Initial antibiotic choices are often based on the most likely pathogen. It is recommended that, following the aspiration of fluid, antibiotics be instilled directly into the vitreous cavity. Intraocular vancomycin, 1 mg, and ceftazidime, 2.25 mg, are frequently used. Amikacin, 400 µg, is used in some centers as an alternative to ceftazidime for gram-negative coverage.

Intravenous antibiotics are considered to have poor penetration into the aqueous humour. Adjunctive therapy with intravenous vancomycin, ceftazidime, and amikacin is frequently employed, although their usefulness remains unclear.

TABLE 16-3. *Endophthalmitis*

Endogenous (septicemic)
  a. Bacillus cereus, candida species, Neisseria meningitidis
Exogenous (direct inoculation)
  a. S. epidermidis, Streptococcus species
Diagnosis
  a. Examination by ophthalmologist
  b. Anterior chamber/vitreous aspiration
  c. Positive gram stain, culture in 60%
Therapy
  a. Intraocular medications
     Vancomycin 1 mg
     Ceftazidine 2.25 mg
     Amikacin 400 μg
  b. Vitrectomy

Ciprofloxacin has been reported to achieve levels above the minimal inhibitory concentration (MIC) for coagulase-negative staphylococcus; some centers use this medication if this pathogen is identified. Intraocular and systemic steroids, in conjunction with vitrectomy, have been used for progressive disease (Table 16.3).

PERITONITIS SECONDARY TO RUPTURED APPENDICITIS

Etiology

Children with appendicitis often have perforation at the time of diagnosis. This perforation leads to the seeding of the peritoneal cavity with the multitude of aerobic and anaerobic organisms found in the gastrointestinal tract. This seeding serves as a risk factor for the development of intra-abdominal abscesses. During recent years, there has been a great interest in the proper management of patients with peritonitis following a perforated appendicitis.

Presentation

Although adults frequently present with periumbilical pain and subsequent migration of point tenderness to the right lower quadrant, up to one half of young children present with the appendicitis already ruptured. These children often present with fever, diffuse abdominal tenderness, and rebound tenderness indicating peritoneal irritation.

Diagnosis

Although the hallmark of infectious disease evaluation is obtaining appropriate cultures, there remains debate about the clinical usefulness of obtaining intraoperative peritoneal cultures in patients with perforated appendicitis. Some studies have demonstrated that culture results do not alter therapy or outcome in patients with peritonitis. This appears to be particularly true when *Pseudomonas aeruginosa* is isolated; in this patient population, *P. aeruginosa* is not considered a clinically important pathogen. Other authors cite alternative studies in which complications were more common in patients whose intraoperative cultures grew an organism that was not covered by the initial antibiotic regimen. One explanation for these discrepancies is that peritoneal cultures are often obtained in children with perforated but not abscessed appendicitis. The potential for abscess formation is extremely low in this population.

Management

In 2003, the Infectious Disease Society of American (IDSA) published guidelines for the selection of antibiotics for complicated intra-abdominal infections. The study reported the clinical usefulness of cultures, particularly in complicated (i.e., those processes associated with peritonitis or abscess formation) intra-abdominal infections. The IDSA recommended that culture and susceptibility be done against the isolated gram-negative bacilli because there is increasing resistance among these organisms. Based on published reports of increasing resistance in the *Bacteroides fragilis* group of organisms, it recommended that empiric use of clindamycin, cefoxitin, and quinolones for treatment of *B. fragilis* **not** be used.

The polymicrobial nature of intra-abdominal infections requires consideration of a broad-spectrum regimen. Coverage against any enteric gram-negative organisms, such as *Escherichia coli,* and anaerobes, such as *Bacteroides* species, is crucial. For this reason, ampicillin, gentamycin, and clindamycin, the traditional "surgical triples," were often used in the past for intra-abdominal infections. As a result of increasing resistance among the gram-negative enteric bacteria and *B. fragilis*, newer regimens are increasingly used. A single combination agent such as ampicillin-sulbactam (Unasyn) or piperacillin-tazobactam (Zosyn), is often used to treat community-acquired intraabdominal infections of mild to moderate severity. Carbapenems, which include imipenem and meropenem, can also be used as single agents because these drugs provide broad-spectrum gram-negative and anaerobic coverage. Combination regimens based on β-lactam antibiotics include third- or fourth-generation cephalosporins such as cefotaxime, ceftriaxone, and cefepime, combined with metronidazole (Flagyl). The latter provides good coverage against *Bacteroides* species, which may be resistant to clindamycin.

Enterococcus is a common organism found in the intestinal tract. In the past, the regimens used to treat complicated intraabdominal infections have provided coverage for this organism. A review of previous studies done by the IDSA found that coverage against enterococci does not provide an advantage and is not necessary in treatment of community-acquired intra-abdominal infection. Similar recommendations can be found for *Candida albicans*, which is isolated in a good percentage of patients who have perforation of the gastrointestinal tract. Unless the patient is re-

TABLE 16-4. *Peritonitis Secondary to Ruptured Appendicitis*

1. Organisms: Polymicrobial including enterococcus, enteric gram negatives (E.coli) and anaerobes (can no longer assume clindamycin susceptibility of Bacteroides fragilis species).
2. Antibiotics for community acquired complicated intra-abdominal infections.
    a. Ampicillin/sulbactam (Unasyn): 100-200 mg/kg/day of ampicillin component divided every six hours.
    b. Piperacilin/ tazobactam (Zosyn): > 6 months ;300-400 mg/kg/day of piperacillin component divided q 6-8 hours.
    c. Imipenem/ cilastin: 15-25 mg/kg every six hours.
    d. Combination regimens: Third or fourth generation cephalosporin: Cefotaxime (100mg/kg/day) in Ceftriaxone (75-100mg/kg/d) or Cefepime (50mg/kg q 8) combined with metronidazole (Flagyl) 30mg/kg/day in 4 divided doses.
3. Children with non-complicated disease, discontinue antibiotics when afebrile and white blood cell counts reveals less than 3% band forms, may also consider changing to oral antibiotics when tolerated to complete ten days therapy.

ceiving immunosuppressive therapy or has recurrent disease, antifungal therapy is not required.

Antibiotic Duration

The duration of antibiotic treatment and the ability to transition to oral antibiotics have also been studied. These studies usually reflect the child with noncomplicated appendicitis in whom there is no extensive infection or abscess in the peritoneal cavity; these are the children most frequently seen by pediatricians. One recent study observed that intravenous antibiotics can be discontinued when the patient is afebrile for 24 hours and the white blood cell count shows less than 3% band forms. Typically, the duration of therapy following this protocol was between 3 and 14 days. Other investigators have evaluated programs in which patients are transitioned to oral amoxicillin-clavulanate (Augmentin) plus metronidazole to complete a 10-day total course. In the patients studied, there was no difference between children who had received oral antibiotic therapy and those who had prolonged intravenous treatment (Table 16.4).

RETROPHARYNGEAL ABSCESS

Etiology

Retropharyngeal abscess is a deep neck infection that can obstruct the upper airway. Most cases occur in patients younger than 5 years of age. These infections are the result of bacteria in the nasopharynx or middle ear infecting the lymph nodes that lie between the posterior pharyngeal wall and the prevertebral fascia. These nodes are thought to atrophy during childhood, which may explain the age distribution seen. Traumatic retropharyngeal abscess is the result of penetrating trauma and can occur at any time in life.

Pathogens

Microbiology of retropharyngeal abscess has been the focus of considerable study. Group A streptococcus is the usual pathogen, although numerous investigators believe there may be a large polymicrobial component. Organisms that have been isolated in children with retropharyngeal abscess include *S. aureus* and anaerobic species such as *Bacteroides* and *Peptostreptococcus* species.

Presentation

Patients often present with a history of sore throat which progresses to increasing neck swelling, drooling, or dysphagia. Affected children may also exhibit decreased neck mobility to such an extent that meningitis is frequently considered and lumbar puncture performed. Increasing stridor has been reported as a classic clinical sign of retropharyngeal abscess, although recent reviews have not found this to be a consistent symptom.

Diagnosis

Diagnosis of retropharyngeal abscess begins with appropriate clinical suspicion in the right clinical setting. Lateral neck films can show an increased retropharyngeal soft tissue space, although interpretation of these plain films may be dependent on patient positioning. Computed tomography of the neck can be extremely helpful in documenting infection in the retropharyngeal space (Fig. 16.2). Evaluation by computed tomography is not without difficulty. There are limitations in the ability of computed tomography to determine definitively whether a well-defined abscess is present; a retropharyngeal cellulitis (or phlegmon) may be difficult to distinguish on computed tomography from a frank abscess. Numerous reports have stated that clinical correlation should be used in making decisions regarding the presence of a true abscess.

Management

Treatment of retropharyngeal cellulitis or abscess always involves the use of appropriate antimicrobials. Ampicillin-sulbactam (Unasyn) offers an advantage in that it has broad-spectrum coverage against not only group A streptococcus and *S. aureus* but also a variety of anaerobic organisms. A combination of clindamycin and a third-generation cephalosporin will also provide coverage for the probable organisms involved. The adjunctive surgical management of retropharyngeal abscess remains controversial. Some reviews and textbooks state that the treatment always includes drainage; many otolaryngologists feel that a trial of antibiotics can be used initially. Failure to respond clinically to medical management alone warrants surgical therapy (Table 16.5).

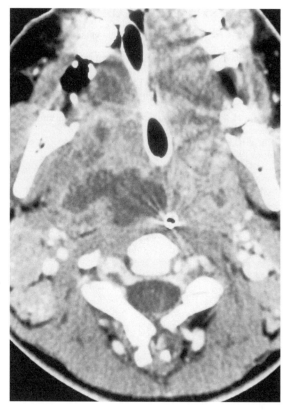

FIG. 16.2. Computed tomography scan revealing
retropharyngeal abscess.

TABLE 16-5. *Retropharyngeal Abscess*

1. Clinical presentation: Fever
   Dysphagia
   Drooling
2. Pathogens: Polymicrobial, including group A streptococci, and oral anaerobes
3. Diagnosis: Computed tomography of neck
4. Antibiotics Clindamycin 20-40 mg/kg/day in 3 divided doses in combination with a
   third generation cephalosporin (cefotaxime or ceftriaxone) or
   unasyn (ampicillin-sulbactam): 100-200 mg/kg/day of ampicillin component in
   4 divided doses
5. Surgery

SELECTED READINGS

Barton LL, Jeck DT, Vaidya VU. Necrotizing fasciitis in children: report of two cases and review of the literature. *Arch Pediatr Adolesc Med* 1996;150(1):105–108.

Brook I. Microbiology of retropharyngeal abscesses in children. *Am J Dis Child* 1987;141(2):202–204.

Craig FW, Schunk JE. Retropharyngeal abscess in children: clinical presentation, utility of imaging, and current management. *Pediatrics* 2003;111(6 Pt 1):1394–1398.

Gollin G, Abarbanell A, Moores D. Oral antibiotics in the management of perforated appendicitis in children. *Am Surg* 2002;68(12):1072–1074.

Hoelzer DJ, Zabel DD, Zern JT. Determining duration of antibiotic use in children with complicated appendicitis. *Pediatr Infect Dis J* 1999;18(11):979–982.

Hsieh WS, Yang PH, Chao HC, et al. Neonatal necrotizing fasciitis: a report of three cases and review of the literature. *Pediatrics* 1999;103(4):E53.

Janssen PA, Selwood BL, Dobson SR, et al. To dye or not to dye: a randomized, clinical trial of a triple dye/alcohol regimen versus dry cord care. *Pediatrics* 2003;111(1):15–20.

Mason WH, Andrews R, Ross LA, et al. Omphalitis in the newborn infant. *Pediatr Infect Dis J* 1989;8(8):521–525.

Solomkin J, Mazuski J, Baron E, et al. Guidelines for the selection of anti-infective agents for complicated intra-abdominal infections. *Clin Infect Dis* 2003;37:997–1005

Vural C, Gungor A, Comerci S. Accuracy of computerized tomography in deep neck infections in the pediatric population. *Am J Otolaryngol* 2003;24:143–148.

Wong CH, Chang CH, Pasupathy S, et al. Necrotizing fasciitis: clinical presentation microbiology, and determinants of mortality. *J Bone Joint Surg Am* 2003;85A(8):1454–1460.

17

Fever and Neutropenia

EPIDEMIOLOGY

Patients undergoing chemotherapy are at considerable risk for serious infection. The primary cell line affected by aggressive chemotherapy is the neutrophil. The absolute neutrophil count (ANC) is calculated by multiplying the total number of white blood cells by the combined percentage of segmented neutrophils and band forms.

A neutrophil count of less than $1,000/m^3$ is frequently associated with serious invasive infection. An absolute neutrophil count of less than $100/m^3$, often seen in patients undergoing chemotherapy, is considered life threatening. The most recent guidelines suggest that **neutropenia** be defined as an absolute neutrophil count of less than $500/m^3$, or less than $1,000/m^3$ if there is the expectation that the counts will decrease to less than $500/m^3$.

ANC = white blood cell count $\times$ % (segmented neutrophils + band forms)

Presentation

Fever in the neutropenic patient is usually defined as a single temperature greater than 38.3°C, (101.3°F) or a sustained temperature of 38°C (100.4°F) temperature for more than 1 hour.

Diagnosis

Due to the risk for life-threatening infection in the patient with fever and neutropenia, current practice suggests that patients meeting the above definitions be admitted to the hospital.

Cultures of the blood, urine, and if possible, induced sputum should be obtained. Chest radiographs are also suggested, especially if respiratory symptoms are present.

Management

The management of the patient with neutropenia and fever can be divided into three major pathogen groups, discussed in the following sections.

GRAM-NEGATIVE BACTERIA IN FEVER AND NEUTROPENIA

In the 1970s, oncology patients were admitted to intensive care centers with fever and neutrophil counts of less than $500/m^3$. It was found that a large number of these patients quickly died from gram-negative sepsis. These gram-negative organisms included *Escherichia coli, Klebsiella* species, and *Enterobacter* species. It was then that the first rule of management of fever and neutropenia was made; the aggressive empiric treatment of gram negative organisms.

Management

To this day, there is no agreement on the optimal gram-negative coverage. Some institutions use double therapy with two separate classes of antibiotics, combining an aminoglycoside and a β-lactam antibiotic such as ceftazidime. Other institutions use monotherapy with a fourth-generation cephalosporin (such as cefepime) or very broad-spectrum combination therapy consisting of imipenem and amikacin. No therapy has proved to be superior. Whatever the regimen used, it is important to realize that gram-negative organisms are the bacteria that cause the patients to expire quickly. A patient with fever and an absolute neutrophil count of less than $1,000/m^3$ is usually admitted with appropriate cultures taken and empirically started on antibiotics effective against gram-negative bacteria.

FUNGAL PATHOGENS IN FEVER AND NEUTROPENIA

The second management principle of fever and neutropenia came about 10 years later. Patients with fever and neutropenia were admitted to the hospital and placed on antibiotics. A number of these patients continued to be febrile with negative blood cultures. A large number of these individuals ultimately died; at autopsy, they were found to have disseminated fungal infection. In the 1980s, results of several large clinical trials suggested that there were fewer fungal infections in persistently febrile neutropenic patients who, after 7 days of fever with negative blood cultures, were given amphotericin B as empiric antifungal therapy. Based on these studies and the autopsy evidence, a patient with fever, neutropenia, and negative blood cultures should have empiric antifungal treatment started after 3 to 7 days; we assume that these patients have fungal infections. The following is a description of the fungal pathogens encountered in the febrile neutropenic patient:

Aspergillus Species

The classic fungal pathogen in the neutropenic oncology patient is *Aspergillus* species. A ubiquitous mold present throughout the environment, aspergillus enters the host by way of the respiratory tract. In the setting of severe qualitative or quantitative neutrophil deficiency, the fungus becomes invasive, resulting in progressive respiratory disease and extrapulmonary dissemination. The common sites of dissemination include the brain, skin, and bone (Figs. 17.1 and 17.2). Progressive sinus disease, pneumonia, and the appearance of new skin or brain lesions should heighten suspicion for aspergillosis in the febrile, neutropenic patient. High-resolution computed tomography (CT) of the chest can be helpful in detecting small nodular lesions, which are common early in the course of invasive aspergillosis.

In recent years, a variety of newer molds have been implicated in severe disease in the neutropenic host. These can present in a fashion similar to aspergillosis, with fever in the setting of continuing neutropenia accompanied by progressive pneumonia, skin lesions, or intracranial lesions. The correct diagnosis of these molds must be confirmed by the isolation in culture because these newer molds may have an initial histologic appearance similar to that of aspergillosis but different antimicrobial sensitivities. These newer molds include the following.

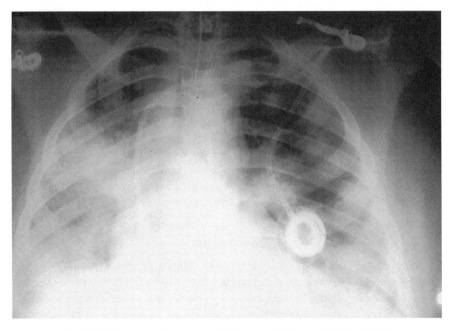

FIG. 17-1. Progressive pneumonia in a child with fever and prolonged neutropenia caused by *Aspergillus* species infection.

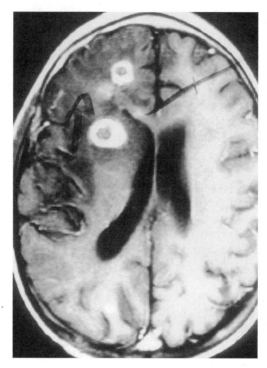

FIG. 17-2. Computed tomography scan of patient with prolonged fever and neutropenia. Cerebral abscess grew *Aspergillus* species.

Fusarium Species

Disseminated disease is common in neutropenic patients, often appearing as painful skin lesions. Unlike other molds, the incidence of positive blood cultures is 50%. Sinusitis and pneumonia are also common. The appearance on biopsy will be similar to that of aspergillus, highlighting the importance of culture diagnosis. *Fusarium* species have a high incidence of *in vitro* amphotericin resistance. Treatment is typically with the newer azole agents such as voriconazole. Surgical débridement of affected areas should be attempted whenever possible.

Zygomycetes

Zygomycetes includes infections with molds *Mucor, Rhizopus, Rhizomucor,* and *Cunninghamella.* They may be differentiated from aspergillosis by their septate hyphae possessing right-angle branching, as opposed to the acute-angle branching seen in aspergillus. Zygomycetes have a predilection for invasion of blood vessels and subsequent dissemination. Rhinocerebral disease is the most common form seen, in which the infection begins in the sinuses and rapidly extends to the orbit and brain. Mucormycosis is typically associated with tissue necrosis and black discoloration; these provide major clues to diagnosis.

Standard treatment for mucormycosis remains amphotericin B. Itraconazole, fluconazole, and voriconazole do not appear useful in treatment of this organism. Adjunctive surgical débridement, with documentation of disease-free margins, is critical for resolution.

Scedosporium Species

When in its sexual state, *Scedosporium* is also known as *Pseudallescheria boydii*. This organism is noteworthy for resistance to most conventional antifungal agents, including an intrinsic amphotericin resistance. *Scedosporium apiospermum*, with its acutely branching hyphae tissue, is similar to aspergillus, stressing the importance of culture in the final identification of any pathogenic mold. Recently, successful treatment has been reported with voriconazole. Surgical débridement should be attempted if at all possible.

Trichosporon Species

Trichosporon asahii, formally referred to as *Trichosporon beigelii*, is increasingly found in neonatal infections and can also be seen in the neutropenic host. *T. asahii* is unusual in that it can be frequently isolated in blood culture. An additional feature of this organism is its ability to cross-react with the capsular polysaccharide of cryptococcus neoformans, resulting in a false-positive latex agglutination test. These fungi have a high frequency of amphotericin resistance and are intrinsically resistant to caspofungin. Therapy with fluconazole has been reported to be successful in the neonatal population.

Diagnosis

Essential to the management of the febrile, neutropenic patient is the establishment of the diagnosis of fungal infection. Certainly, not every patient with fever and neutropenia has a fungal infection. Polymerase chain reaction (PCR) testing against genetic sequences of *Candida* and *Aspergillus* species has been used to detect evolving fungal infection in febrile neutropenic hosts. Preliminary reports suggest that this is a sensitive method and in the future may help define the patient population that can most benefit from antifungal therapy. Galactomannan is a polysaccharide component of the fungal wall that has recently been approved as a method for early detection of invasive aspergillosis. An enzyme-linked immunoabsorbent assay (ELISA) has been developed, and serial evaluations of this component in neutropenic hosts may be useful in detecting evolving invasive aspergillosis. The test uses an optical density index; a positive result in the United States is greater than or equal to 0.5. It should be stressed that a single negative test does not rule out evolving aspergillosis. Serial evaluations in conjunction with clinical, radiographic, and culture examinations are always necessary.

Management

Traditionally, the gold standard antifungal agent has been amphotericin B. The traditional form of amphotericin B is amphotericin B deoxycholate. The dose given is 0.6 to 1.0 mg/kg per day. Although progressive dosing over several days has been tried in the past, many clinicians believe this is no longer necessary and delays the administration of an appropriate dose. There are now three lipid-associated formulations of amphotericin B: amphotericin B lipid complex (Abelcet), amphotericin B colloidal dispersion (Amphotec), and liposomal amphotericin B (AmBisome). There is still no definitive evidence that these newer formulations are actually better antifungal agents. There is some evidence that these newer agents may decrease the metabolic or renal complications seen with amphotericin B deoxycholate. Some clinicians use the lipid-associated amphotericin preparations as front-line agents in patients with a higher risk for nephrotoxicity or renal failure (i.e., additional concurrent nephrotoxic drugs, history of underlying renal disease). If these are to be used, it is important that the practitioner realize that the dosing is different. The dosing of the lipid and liposomal formulations is 3 to 5 mg/kg per day.

Newer Antifungal Agents

A common question is the role of newer antifungal agents in the management of neutropenic fever in the oncology unit. Fluconazole (Diflucan) is readily available and is often well tolerated; the major disadvantage is that it lacks activity against *Aspergillus* species, a major pathogen in this patient population. Some investigators have attempted to define the use of a particular antifungal based on the duration of neutropenia. Yeasts, usually *Candida* species, are common early in the course of neutropenia. Molds, such as *Aspergillus* species, usually are seen in the second week of a low neutrophil count. The use of fluconazole for treatment of fever and neutropenia should be discouraged in patients who have been on long-term fungal prophylaxis because these patients are known to have an increased risk for infection with fluconazole-resistant isolates (such as *Candida krusei* and *Candida glabrata*). In addition, fluconazole should not be used if a patient has progressive sinus or pulmonary disease consistent with an *Aspergillus* species infection.

Several additional agents have been developed to treat disseminated fungus in the immunocompromised host. Intravenous itraconazole is an azole that has activity against *Aspergillus* species. Response rates are similar to other agents; concerns about potential drug interactions at the cytochrome P450 level can limit use. Recently, the U.S. Food and Drug Administration (FDA) has licensed caspofungin (Cancidas), which belongs to a new class of drugs called echinocandins. This drug is indicated for patients with invasive aspergillosis that is nonresponsive to amphotericin. Early studies report a salvage rate of 40%. Caspofungin is also effective for candidemia and invasive candidiasis and has FDA approval for these indications. Voriconazole (Vfend) has recently been approved and offers the advantage of good *Aspergillus* species coverage, good cerebrospinal fluid penetration, and coverage against some of the newer molds affecting cancer patients. Studies comparing voriconazole versus amphotericin B have found it a suitable alternative for empiric antifungal treatment in patients with fever and neutropenia. In the future, these drugs, either alone or in combination, may represent a major advantage in antifungal therapy in the neutropenic patient.

Fungi and Mold Seen in Fever and Neutropenia

Organism	Comment
Candida species	Sensitive to fluconazole, with exception of *C. krusei* and *C. glabrata*
Aspergillus species	Resistant to fluconazole
	Sensitive to amphotericin, itraconazole, voriconazole, caspofungin
Fusarium species	High incidence of *in vitro* amphotericin resistance
	Voriconazole reported effective
	Surgical débridement often needed
Scedosporium species	Intrinsic amphotericin resistance
	Voriconazole reported affective
	Surgical débridement often needed
Trichosporon species	High frequency of amphotericin resistance
	Intrinsically resistant to caspofungin
Zygomycetes	
Mucor species	Resistant to itraconazole, voriconazole
Rhizopus species	Amphotericin, sensitive surgical débridement often needed

GRAM-POSITIVE PATHOGENS IN FEVER AND NEUTROPENIA

In the 1990s, a new chapter was added to the management of fever and neutropenia. The emergence of infections with gram-positive organisms was seen in oncology centers across the country. Currently, up to 60% of the bacteria isolated from blood cultures of febrile children with cancer are now gram-positive organisms. A gram-positive organism frequently isolated is the α-hemolytic streptococcus (AHS). This includes a diverse group of streptococci, such as *Streptococcus mitis*, *Streptococcus sanguis*, and *Streptococcus milleri*. When isolated from blood culture, these bacteria are often identified as α-hemolytic or viridans streptococci rather than a specific species designation. These organisms are part of the normal oral flora and are also part of the flora of the gastrointestinal tract. They are thought to enter the bloodstream and become invasive following the breakdown of oral and gastrointestinal mucosa that accompanies chemotherapy. There are several risk factors associated with viridans streptococcal bacteremia in febrile neutropenic patients; these include oral mucositis, acute myelogenous leukemia, and high-dose cytosine arabinoside therapy.

It is also appreciated that viridans streptococcal bacteremia in patients with profound neutropenia can be associated with a variety of severe life-threatening complications. A syndrome similar to toxic shock syndrome characterized by hypotension, rash, and the development of acute respiratory distress syndrome (ARDS) has been seen in up to one fourth of neutropenic patients with AHS bacteremia. Progression to severe hypotension and respiratory failure can occur despite rapid clearance of bacteria from the bloodstream. The mechanism of this severe syndrome is not understood, although it may involve production of toxins.

Management

A major concern is that antibiotic resistance among AHS is increasing. Although studies are limited, it is found that up to half of the isolates showed at least intermediate resistance to penicillin, defined as a minimal inhibitory concentration (MIC) of 0.25 to 2.0 µg/mL. In addition, centers have reported that more than 50% of AHS show at least intermittent resistance to ceftazidime, defined as an MIC of more than 1.0 µg/mL.

The emergence of the gram-positive infections in patients with cancer has led to a discussion whether vancomycin should be used as initial empiric therapy in the management of fever and neutropenia. Early studies showed that the initial use of vancomycin in patients with fever and neutropenia did not significantly alter outcome. Recent studies have shown that, although this may be true for gram-positive organisms taken as a whole, there is evidence that the early use of vancomycin can produce a survival advantage in specific cases of AHS infection. Patients who ultimately were diagnosed with AHS infection who received empiric vancomycin had a significantly improved outcome over that of patients whose vancomycin was delayed until final identification of the infecting organism. It may be that vancomycin does become a part of initial empiric treatment for fever and neutropenia in children, especially if specific risk factors are present (Table 17.1). If empiric treatment is initiated with vancomycin, it should be discontinued once culture specimens fail to reveal gram-positive organisms.

TABLE 17.1. *Antimicrobials Used in Pediatric Fever and Neutropenia*

1. Initial treatment: gram-negative coverage
   a. Tobramycin, 6–7.5 mg/kg/d divided q6–8h, in combination with ceftazidime (Fortaz), 50 mg/kg IV q8h
   b. Cefepime (Maxipime), 50 mg/kg IV q8h
   c. Imipenem/cilastatin (Primaxin), 15–25 mg/kg q6h
2. Persistent fever, neutropenia with negative blood cultures
   a. Amphotericin B deoxycholate, 0.6 mg/kg/d
   a. Lipid formulation amphotericin (Abelcet), 3–5 mg/kg/d
   b. Liposomal formulation amphotericin (AmBisome), 3–5 mg/kg/d
   c. Voriconazole (Vfend)—dose recommended for children older than 12 years: 6 mg/kg IV q12h for two doses, then 4 mg/kg q12h
   d. Caspofungin (Cancidas). Pediatric dose not established. Adults receive 70 mg IV ×1, then 50 mg/d thereafter.
3. Consideration for initial vancomycin use (15–20 mg/kg IV q12h)
   a. Hypotension
   b. In-dwelling catheter
   c. Severe mucositis
   d. Acute myelogenous leukemia

DURATION OF THERAPY IN FEVER AND NEUTROPENIA

A major issue in managing the oncology patient with fever is the duration of therapy. There are several possibilities when managing this patient population, usually determined by the recovery of the neutrophil count.

Patient Afebrile within the First 3 to 5 Days of Treatment, Etiology Found

If a responsible pathogen is isolated, the antibiotics can be changed to give optimal treatment to the specific pathogen. Antibiotic treatment should be continued for a minimum of 7 days; many specialists continue treatment for at least 10 to 14 days if an isolate is recovered in blood culture. Often, antibiotics are continued until there is evidence of bone marrow recovery (i.e., neutrophil count > $500/m^3$). In cases in which neutropenia is predicted to be prolonged, afebrile patients may have antibiotics stopped and are closely observed.

Patient Afebrile, No Etiology Found

The management of these patients is difficult because no infectious disease process has been documented. Patients who are afebrile and who have an absolute neutrophil count of more than $500/m^3$ may have their antibiotics discontinued. In persistently neutropenic children, there has been an effort to divide patients into low-risk and high-risk categories. Children are considered at low risk if they lack ongoing signs of sepsis, chills, hypotension, severe mucositis, and have a neutrophil count of more than $100/m^3$. In these children, antibiotics may be stopped when the child is afebrile for about 1 week. A small number of studies have suggested that the antibiotic can be changed to oral cefixime and the child monitored closely. It should be noted that these studies involving the use of oral antibiotics often took place with the patients remaining as inpatients for close monitoring. Children who are labeled at high risk (i.e., those with continued absolute neutropenia or mucositis, or in whom follow-up cannot be guaranteed) are continued on intravenous antibiotics until the resolution of neutropenia.

Continued Fever without Etiology

Patients who continue to have fever without obvious etiology present the most difficult management dilemma. The most important management principal in these patients is continued evaluation with physical examination, blood cultures, and radiographic studies. Because systemic fungal infections can be associated with negative blood cultures and may present with progressive intracranial, sinus, or pulmonary disease, these areas should be closely monitored. Examination of the oropharynx for viral lesions caused by either herpes simplex virus or cytomegalovirus is important. Children with persistent fever and neutropenia are often treated for 2 weeks, with a complete reevaluation at that time. In certain situations, it has been suggested that if the patient remains clinically stable with no evidence of progressive infectious disease, antibiotics may be discontinued under close observation.

SPECIFIC CLINICAL ENTITIES IN FEVER AND NEUTROPENIA

Hepatosplenic Candidiasis

Etiology

An important clinical entity in the patient with fever and neutropenia is hepatosplenic candidiasis. Hepatosplenic candidiasis represents a disseminated candidal infection, with the liver and spleen being the primary sites affected. All species of candida have been reported to cause this condition. The major risk factor is prolonged neutropenia. Of note, most affected patients become symptomatic only after recovery of their neutrophil count.

Presentation

Patients present with persistent fever and abdominal distention and pain. Blood cultures, as in the case of most fungal infections in this patient population, remain negative. Patients often have elevated transaminase and alkaline phosphatase levels.

Diagnosis

Diagnosis is by CT or magnetic resonance imaging of the abdomen, which shows numerous hepatosplenic lesions. Biopsy of these lesions is positive in more than 80% of cases.

Management

Treatment is prolonged antifungal therapy. Antifungal treatment should continue until there is radiographic resolution of lesions.

Typhlitis

Etiology

Typhlitis is also known as **neutropenic enterocolitis**. Often localized to the cecum, it is associated with profound neutropenia in a patient with underlying malignancy. Affected patients often have absolute neutropenia, fever, abdominal pain, and distention. Gastrointestinal bleeding is frequently seen. The pathogenesis of typhlitis remains unknown. Chemotherapy is thought to damage the mucosa of the bowel and predispose it to bacterial overgrowth injury. Bacterial overgrowth can lead to invasion of the mucosa and even breakthrough bacteremia. A variety of pathogens have been cultured from the blood in patients with typhlitis, including *Pseudomonas* species, *Staphylococcus aureus*, enteric gram-negative organisms, anaerobes, and viridans streptococci. Fungal pathogens are also thought to be involved in the pathogenesis of typhlitis; common isolates include *Candida* and *Aspergillus* species.

Presentation

Patients with typhlitis typically have a history of prolonged neutropenia. Abdominal pain and distention are prominent symptoms.

Diagnosis

Definitive diagnosis requires biopsy of the bowel, which shows focal hemorrhage, ulceration, and intramural edema. Because physicians are often reluctant to perform bowel biopsy in a patient so critically ill, CT has been increasingly used in patients with suspected typhlitis. Findings on CT include thickening of the bowel and accumulation of peritoneal fluid.

Management

Management of typhlitis includes intensive supportive care, including parenteral nutrition. It is traditional that broad-spectrum antimicrobial agents be given to such patients, including antibiotics with efficacy against resistant gram-negative organisms, AHS, and fungi. Surgical management is done in extreme cases, although most surgeons believe that patients who require surgery for typhlitis face a very grim prognosis. Resolution of underlying neutropenia is a major factor in recovery.

SELECTED READINGS

Elting LS, Rubenstein EB, Rolston K, et al. Outcome of bacteremia in patients with cancer and neutropenia: observation from two decades of epidemiological and clinical trials. *Clin Infect Dis* 1997;25(2):247–259.

Hughes WT, Armstrong D, Bodey GP, et al. 2002 Guidelines for the use of antimicrobial agents in neutropenic patients with cancer. *Clin Infect Dis* 2002;34(6):730–751.

Katz JA, Wagner ML, Gresik MV, et al. Typhlitis: an 18 year experience and post-mortem review. *Cancer* 1990;65(4):1041–1047.

Kauffman CA. Fungal infections. *Infect Med* 2003;20:424–436.

Sallah S, Semelka RC, Wehbie R, et al. Hepatosplenic candidiasis in patients with acute leukaemia. *Br J Haematol* 1999;106(3):697–701.

Tunkel AR, Sepkowitz KA. Infections caused by viridans streptococci in patients with neutropenia. Clin Infect Dis 2002;34(11):1524–1529.

Walsh TJ, Pappas P, Winston D. et al. Voriconazole compared with liposomal amphotericin B for empirical antifungal therapy in patients with neutropenia and persistent Fever. *N Engl of Med* 2002;346(4):225–234.

18

Fever of Unknown Origin

EPIDEMIOLOGY

In the early 1960s, fever of unknown origin (FUO) was defined in adults as fever lasting longer than 3 weeks with no obvious diagnosis after 1 week of inpatient evaluation. A variety of definitions have subsequently been used to define FUO in children, ranging from 2 to 3 weeks of unexplained fever, with at least 1 week being an inpatient evaluation. Many investigators have settled on the following definition: a normal host with oral or rectal temperature greater than 38°C (100.4°F) at least twice a week for more than 3 weeks. It is important at the outset to make the distinction between FUO and the more common **fever without localizing signs,** defined as fever for less than 2 weeks' duration. The latter is relatively common in children and is usually caused by a viral illness.

Categories of Pediatric Fever of Unknown Origin

1. Infectious
2. Malignancies
3. Rheumatologic disorders

Etiologies of pediatric FUO have changed during the past three decades. Recent studies suggest that as many as 50% of children who present with prolonged fever resolve their fever without determination of cause; this is in contrast to the 10% to 20% of patients who had resolution of fever without a diagnosis 20 to 30 years ago. It has been suggested that the increased percentage of undiagnosed cases is the result of advances in laboratory and radiographic testing that diagnose major infections and malignancies earlier. It is thought that most prolonged fevers in children that resolve without definitive diagnosis are the result of viral infections that are difficult to diagnose. The major issue in evaluating a child with FUO is to identify those children who have a potentially treatable infectious, malignant, or rheumatologic condition.

The evaluation of a child with FUO can be a considerable challenge given the extensive differential diagnosis involved. There are several recommended approaches; the first is to consider the specific organ systems often involved in prolonged fever.

INFECTIOUS CAUSES

Specific Areas associated with Pediatric Fever of Unknown Origin

Respiratory. Sinusitis is often reported to be a cause of low-grade, prolonged fever. Because sinus aspiration is not done routinely, upper respiratory infection symptoms that last longer than 2 weeks provide the major clue for bacterial sinus infection.
Dental. Careful examination should always be done, evaluating for dental caries and abscess formation.
Urinary tract. This is a common cause of prolonged fever in children. Young children may not complain of dysuria but rather of abdominal pain and anorexia. Many children with prolonged fever receive a chest x-ray, numerous blood tests, and never have urinary tract infection considered. A certain percentage of urinary tract infections are missed on dipstick testing and even urinalysis. If urinary tract infection is considered, culture and sensitivity tests of an appropriately obtained urine specimen should be done.
Pneumonia. Lower respiratory infection is common in children and may be associated with increased respiratory rate, increased work of breathing, and hypoxia. A chest radiograph is often considered a front-line study in patients with prolonged fever.

Pediatric FUO can also be approached by considering not only specific areas of infection but also unusual bacteria associated with prolonged fever. The following list is a summary of some unusual pathogens involved in pediatric FUO.

Unusual Bacteria associated with Pediatric Fever of Unknown Origin

Cat-scratch disease. Exposure to kittens or cats is frequently elicited. Classically described as causing lymphadenopathy, this infection is increasingly described as a cause of pediatric FUO. It can be associated with a granulomatous hepatitis, which can be seen by computed tomography. Diagnosis is by serology showing the causative agent, *Bartonella henselae*.
Brucellosis. *Brucella* species are gram-negative coccobacilli. Disease is caused by exposure to unpasteurized dairy products and in some areas is a major cause of prolonged fever. Travelers to endemic areas may not be aware of exposure through regional foods. Patients can present with fever, arthralgias, hepatosplenomegaly, and orchitis. Diagnosis is by serology and by culture of the bacteria from blood or bone marrow. If brucellosis is suspected, blood cultures must be held for at least 21 days due to slow growth of the organism.

Tuberculosis. This is seen in patients traveling to endemic areas or who have family members visiting from endemic areas. Miliary disease can present with prolonged fever and weight loss. Early on, miliary disease on chest x-ray may not be readily appreciated, and sequential films may be required if the diagnosis is suspected. A tuberculin skin test should also be done in all patients suspected of having tuberculosis.

Malaria. Patients present with spiking fevers, anemia, and splenomegaly. The diagnosis is made by examination of both thin and thick smears of the blood looking for malaria parasites. The thick smears are made by applying blood twice to a slide; these smears contain more red blood cells to examine for parasites. Identification of the actual species of malaria is often easier to determine on thin smears. Therapy for malaria depends on the infecting species.

Salmonella. Enteric fever refers to invasive *Salmonella* species infection. The most common enteric fever is that caused by *Salmonella typhi* species. After ingestion, the invasive salmonella enters the bloodstream from the gastrointestinal tract. Diarrhea may not be a principal symptom because the organism does not reside long in the gastrointestinal tract. The diagnosis is suggested by high fevers, leukopenia, organomegaly, and an embolic rash (rose spots). Diagnosis is by blood culture. Because enteric fever is one of the major treatable forms of FUO, in the correct epidemiologic setting, it should always be considered (see Chapter 14).

Rickettsial disease. This is a group of tick-borne illnesses, which are obligate intracellular pathogens. The major rickettsial disease is Rocky Mountain spotted fever (RMSF), characterized by fever, headache, and an extremity rash. Its cause is *Rickettsia rickettsii.*

RMSF is found throughout the United States and is transmitted by a tick bite. The spring and summer months are the months of highest incidence. States with the highest incidence of RMSF include North Carolina and Oklahoma, although a large number of cases are reported in Arkansas, Tennessee, and Missouri. The rash of RMSF may begin as a macular exanthem, which then becomes petechial. Typical distribution is on the wrists and ankles, with spread to the trunk. The distribution of the exanthem on the palms and soles provides a major clue to the diagnosis.

The diagnosis of RMSF is established by serology, usually an indirect immunofluorescence antibody (IFA). Patients with an exposure history and clinical presentation compatible with RMSF should have empiric treatment given. The drug of choice is doxycycline, even though this drug is typically not given to children younger than 8 years of age.

Ehrlichiosis includes human monocytic ehrlichiosis (HME) and human granulocytic ehrlichiosis (HGE). HME occurs in the southeastern and south central United States, whereas HGE is reported in Wisconsin, Minnesota, Connecticut, and New York, as well as the West Coast. Ehrlichiosis is a febrile illness that is similar to RMSF but is less frequently associated with rash. Leukopenia, anemia, and hepatitis are frequent findings. Diagnosis is by serology. Doxycycline is again the treatment of choice. The rickettsial diseases highlight the importance of a history regarding tick exposure and travel.

Dengue. Dengue fever is an arboviral infection associated with fever, myalgia, leukopenia, and rash. Dengue virus is transmitted by mosquito vectors. Dengue is found primarily in tropical areas, particularly the Caribbean and Central and South America. Dengue hemorrhagic fever is considered the most severe of the spectrum, and it is thought to be caused by repeated infections by a variety of dengue serotypes. Diagnosis is by serology. Treatment is supportive.

Leptospirosis. Leptospira are spirochetes typically found in animals. This illness results from exposure to water that has been contaminated with the urine of dogs, rats, and livestock. Exposure can occur by exposure to fresh water or to occupational work with animals. Patients who participate in freshwater sports while on vacation are at risk for the disease. Acute leptospirosis can manifest as fever, myalgias, jaundice, and conjunctival redness. Laboratory evaluation may reveal aseptic meningitis and elevation of the liver function tests. Diagnosis is by blood and cerebrospinal fluid cultures, although the organism is difficult to grow. Serology is available and is usually the method used for diagnosis.

Rat-bite fever. Rat bite fever is caused by either of two organisms: *Streptobacillus moniliformis* or *Spirillum minus*. The disease is transmitted by the bite of rats, ingestion of contaminated food products, or contact with an infected animal. Patients present with high fever, a maculopapular or petechial rash (predominantly on the extremities), arthralgias, and arthritis. Diagnosis is by culture of the organism; anaerobic blood cultures or the use of special media may be required. Treatment is with intravenous penicillin.

Relapsing fever. This illness is caused by the spirochete *Borrelia recurrentis*; patients present with high fever, arthralgia, and often a macular rash of the trunk. Infection is caused by tick exposure in western mountainous areas and national parks. The first febrile episode is followed by a period of wellness with one or more relapses, which become progressively shorter. Diagnosis is made by eliciting an exposure history and viewing a spirochete on a peripheral blood smear. Treatment is with penicillin, doxycycline, or erythromycin.

Viral Infections associated with Fever of Unknown Origin

Adenovirus infection is often associated with pharyngitis or conjunctivitis. The conjunctivitis can be hemorrhagic associated with a pseudomembrane. The diagnosis can be made by serology or by a viral culture of eyes or nasopharynx.

Mononucleosis syndrome (Epstein-Barr virus and cytomegalovirus). These viral pathogens produce a syndrome often associated with elevated liver function tests, rash, and pharyngitis. Diagnosis is by serology.

Hepatitis. Hepatitis viruses A, B, and occasionally C can present with prolonged fever. In the younger child, these conditions may be anicteric. Initial suspicion will be made by organomegaly and elevation of the liver function tests. Diagnosis is by serology.

Kawasaki Disease

Kawasaki disease is an inflammatory condition of unknown etiology occurring predominantly in children younger than 5 years of age. Although an infectious cause is not proved, it should be considered in the differential diagnosis of prolonged fever in children.

Kawasaki disease is a clinical diagnosis in which the criteria are as follows:

1. Fever for longer than 5 days.
2. Erythematous mouth with strawberry tongue and red, cracked lips.
3. A polymorphous rash that can be morbilliform, maculopapular, or erythema multiforme.
4. Swollen hands and feet.
5. Unilateral cervical adenitis.
6. Bulbar conjunctivitis without exudate.

Additional signs seen in Kawasaki disease include elevation of liver function tests, peripheral facial nerve palsy, sterile pyuria, aseptic meningitis, and hydrops of the gallbladder.

The major concern is that untreated Kawasaki disease will result in coronary artery aneurysms in about 20% of cases. Treatment is with intravenous immunoglobulin at a dose of 2 g/kg given over 10 to 12 hours. Additional treatment involves aspirin at high dose of 80 to 100 mg/kg in four divided doses for several days while fever resolves. Subsequently, aspirin is given at a dose of 3 to 5 mg/kg per day once a day for 6 to 8 weeks until the sedimentation rate and platelet count are normal.

There is increasing appreciation that infants younger than 6 months of age may have Kawasaki disease without having all clinical criteria necessary for diagnosis. It is concerning because these same young infants have a high incidence of subsequent coronary artery aneurysm formation. The term "atypical" or "incomplete" Kawasaki disease is currently used to describe children, typically young infants, who fail to meet the criteria for Kawasaki disease but have no other explanation for their clinical course and laboratory findings. Infants usually have persistent fever, extremely high sedimentation rate and C-reactive protein, and increasing platelet counts.

Kawasaki disease is typically seen in the first 5 years of life and should always be considered in children with prolonged fever. Although some cases of Kawasaki disease have all criteria manifesting at once, in many cases, the clinical manifestations have sequential appearance. When taking a history in a child with FUO, one should always specifically ask about swollen hands, conjunctivitis, and the appearance of rashes (Table 18.1).

TABLE 18.1. *Specific Infections associated with Pediatric Fever of Unknown Origin*

Infections	Clinical Features	Diagnosis
Tuberculosis (*Mycobacterium tuberculosis*)	Weight loss	Tuberculin skin test; chest x-ray
Malaria (*Plasmodium* species)	Hepatosplenomegaly Travel to endemic region	Thick smears of peripheral blood
Cat-scratch disease (*Bartonella henselae*)	Cat exposure Organomegaly Granulomatous lesions (seen on abdominal computed tomography scan)	Serology Biopsy
Salmonella species (including *S. typhi*)	Diarrhea Organomegaly, "rose spots" Leukopenia	Blood culture Stool culture
Brucella species (*B. canis, B. abortus*)	Arthralgias Exposure to unpasteurized dairy products	Serology
Rat-bite fever (*Streptobacillus moniliformis, Spirillum minus*)	Exposure to rats Pustular rash on palms, soles Arthritis	Blood culture
Viral pathogens		
Epstein-Barr virus	Rash, tonsillitis, hepatitis	Serology
Cytomegalovirus	Rash, hepatitis	Serology
Adenovirus	Conjunctivitis	Serology
Borrelia recurrentis	Relapsing fever	Thick smears of peripheral blood
Kawasaki disease	Fever greater than 5 days Conjunctivitis (bulbar) Cervical adenopathy (unilateral) Swollen hands and feet Rash (polymorphous) Mucous membrane erythema, cracked lips	
Leptospirosis	Dog exposure Aseptic meningitis	Culture Serology

NONINFECTIOUS CAUSES

In addition to the infectious differential diagnosis, the clinician should be aware of the major noninfectious causes of pediatric FUO.

Systemic Lupus Erythematosus

Systemic lupus erythematosus (SLE) is an inflammatory condition of unknown etiology. The inflammation can affect virtually any organ system, including the skin, kidneys, and central nervous system. Criteria for the diagnosis of SLE have been revised. Often, the presentation will include prolonged fever. Symptoms relating to SLE, such as alopecia, oral ulcers, and arthritis, should be part of the evaluation, particularly in high-risk populations such as teenaged girls.

Diagnosis

Criteria for Diagnosis of SLE

Four of the following criteria are required for diagnosis:
1. Malar rash
2. Arthritis
3. Discoid rash
4. Antinuclear antibody (ANA)
5. Serositis
   a. Pericardial disease
   b. Pleural effusion
6. Oral ulcers
7. Neurologic disorder (seizures, psychosis)
8. Leukopenia, thrombocytopenia, hemolytic anemia
9. Renal disease
10. Photosensitivity
11. Autoantibody (anti-DNA, anti-Sm, false-positive VDRL)

Systemic Juvenile Rheumatoid Arthritis

Although it is the least common form of juvenile rheumatoid arthritis, pediatricians often see children with the systemic form because they frequently present with prolonged fever. The classic presentation is twice-daily fevers in which baseline temperature rises then falls below normal. Extreme elevation of sedimentation rate, often greater than 100 mm/h, is common. Other laboratory findings include leukocytosis, increased liver function tests, and a decreased serum albumin. Polyarthritis may not be evident for weeks to months after disease onset.

Systemic juvenile rheumatoid arthritis is thought to be a diagnosis of exclusion and is considered only after a complete diagnostic examination, including bone marrow evaluation.

Malignancy

Always a concern in a patient with prolonged fever is the possibility of cancer. The major cancers in the pediatric population include leukemia, lymphomas, and neuroblastoma. Particular attention should be paid to the presence of pallor, bruising, progressive adenopathy (particularly in the supraclavicular area), and hepatosplenomegaly.

The possibility of an underlying malignancy causing prolonged fever is a source of great anxiety to both caretakers and clinicians. In addition to history and clinical exam, certain laboratory markers can be helpful in identifying those children with a malignancy. In addition to marked elevation of the sedimentation rate, serum uric acid and lactate dehydrogenase levels are often elevated.

DIAGNOSTIC EVALUATION OF THE CHILD WITH FEVER OF UNKNOWN ORIGIN

History

The medical evaluation begins with a precise determination of duration and character of the fever, travel history, animal exposure, and associated illness in family members.

Specifics of the history should include the following:

- Duration and characteristics of the fever (number of spikes per day, timing of the temperature elevation, whether the temperature returns to normal or below normal)
- Travel history or exposure to people who have traveled to regions endemic for particular diseases (typhoid, malaria, tuberculosis, RMSF)
- Exposure to any animals (cat-scratch disease, rat-bite fever, leptospirosis)
- Exposure to unpasteurized dairy products (brucellosis)
- Presence of rashes, conjunctivitis, mucous membrane changes, and arthritis (juvenile arthritis, Kawasaki syndrome, SLE)
- Presence of associated cough, weight loss, or lymphadenopathy (lymphoma, leukemia, neuroblastoma)
- Specific complaints (abdominal pain, arthritis, chronic headache)

Physical Examination

The physical examination should always be done keeping in mind the possible entities that were elicited from the history. Sequential examination may be necessary; one group of investigators found that repeated physical examinations led to the diagnosis in more than one half of cases. Each organ system should be examined as it relates to the particular processes that are possible in a child with pediatric FUO.

Skin: Presence of rashes, areas of desquamation, photosensitivity, and vasculitic lesions
Eyes: Conjunctivitis
Mucous membranes: ulcerations, redness, dental caries, and oral thrush
Lymphatic: Adenopathy in cervical, supraclavicular, and axillary regions
Cardiac: murmurs, gallops, friction rubs
Abdomen: Hepatosplenomegaly, tenderness
Extremities: Presence of arthritis, swollen hands and feet
Neurologic: Orientation, mental status

Laboratory Evaluation

Laboratory evaluation of the child with prolonged fever is often divided into several steps.

Step 1 often includes the following:

- Sedimentation rate
- Complete blood count with differential (evaluation for anemia, thrombocytopenia, presence of blasts)
- Metabolic panel, including BUN, creatinine, liver function tests, lactate dehydrogenase, and uric acid levels
- Urinalysis and urine culture
- Chest x-ray and tuberculin skin test
- Epstein-Barr virus and cytomegalovirus serology
- Viral culture of the nasopharynx and eyes (if clinically warranted)
- Specific serology as suggested by the history or risk factors

Step 2 of the evaluation is always dictated by the history and repeated physical examination. Step 2 is more invasive and can include the following:

Echocardiogram. Evaluate for coronary artery brightness or aneurysms associated with Kawasaki disease and pericardial effusion associated with various rheumatologic conditions, including SLE.

Abdominal or pelvic computed tomography. Detection of occult abscesses or granulomatous lesions

Bone scan. Evaluation for occult osteomyelitis or discitis

Serology. As clinically indicated by history or physical exam

ANA, double-stranded DNA, compliment levels (if history or physical suggests SLE)

Although a variety of scanning procedures, including computed tomography and radionucleotide scans, are often obtained in patients with FUO, it has been reported that these studies usually do not lead to a diagnosis not previously suspected by the history or physical examination. Indications for scanning for occult abscess, granuloma lesions, or infiltrative diseases should always be based on the history and clinical examination.

Step 3 is considered the most invasive step and can include the following:

- Bone marrow aspiration, looking for infiltrative process or to culture a variety of organisms (such as brucellosis, tuberculosis, or disseminated fungal infection).
- Biopsy of suspicious skin lesions or lymph nodes.
- Endoscopy and biopsy

As many as one half of patients with prolonged FUO do not receive a definitive diagnosis. The clinician must decide, based on the individual patient, which treatable processes need to be considered. It has been suggested that, once this has been done, the patient may be monitored closely. A period of 4 to 5 weeks has been reported as an acceptable duration for prolonged fever once serious pathology has been ruled out.

Management

TABLE 18.2. *Management of Major Infections Associated with Pediatric Fever of Unknown Origin*

Disease	Treatment
1. Cat-scratch disease	a. Lymphadenopathy: azithromycin, 10 mg/kg/d for 1 d followed by 5 mg/kg/d for 4 days; needle aspiration b. Disseminated disease: azithromycin may be required for several months
2. Tuberculosis	a. Multidrug treatment Isoniazid, 10 mg/kg/d Rifampin, 15 mg/kg/d Pyrazinamide, 20–40 mg/kg/d Ethambutol, 15 mg/kg/d
3. Brucellosis	a. Doxycycline, 200 mg/d in 2 divided doses, or trimethoprim-sulfamethoxazole (Bactrim), 10 mg/kg/d of trimethoprim component in 2 divided doses; treatment often required for 4–6 wk b. Rifampin, 15–20 mg/kg/d in 1 or 2 divided doses, often recommended for combination therapy
4. *Salmonella typhi* infection (invasive or enteric fever)	a. Cefotaxime, 100–200 mg/kg/d in 3 divided doses; or ceftriaxone, 50–75 mg/kg/d in 1 or 2 doses b. Ciprofloxacin, ampicillin can be used if sensitivities dictate c. Treatment usually given for 10–14 d
5. Rocky Mountain spotted fever	a. Doxycycline >45 kg: 5 mg/kg/d in 2 divided doses <45 kg: 100 mg/PO twice daily b. Treatment usually given for 7 d
6. Leptospirosis	a. Penicillin G, 100,000–400,000 U/kg/24 hr in 4 divided doses b. Doxycycline for patients older than 8 yr
7. Rat-bite fever	a. Penicillin G, 100,000–400,000 U/kg/24 hr in 4 divided doses b. Procaine penicillin IM, 25,000–50,000 U/Kg/d in 2 divided doses c. Treatment usually given for 7 d
8. Relapsing fever	a. Penicillin G, 100, 000–400,000 U/kg/d in 4 divided doses b. Treatment usually given for 7 d
9. Kawasaki disease	a. Intravenous immune globulin (IVIG), 2 g/kg/dose ×1 b. Aspirin, 80–100 mg/kg/d in 4 divided doses until fever resolves, then 3–5 mg/kg/d until platelets and sedimentation rate are normal

PERIODIC FEVER

> When taking a history for FUO, it is important to distinguish FUO from periodic fever.

Whereas FUO implies a more continuous process, **periodic fever** is defined as three or more episodes of fever in a 6-month period with an interval of at least 7 days between febrile episodes. There are several classic periodic fever syndromes with which the general pediatrician should be familiar.

PFAPA Syndrome

Etiology

PFAPA is the syndrome of periodic fever, aphthous ulcers, pharyngitis, and adenitis. This is the most common periodic fever syndrome in pediatrics. Its etiology remains unknown. It is usually found in children younger than 5 years of age.

Presentation

The PFAPA syndrome is characterized by periodic episodes of high fevers lasting 3 to 6 days with recurrence every 21 to 28 days. Patients often have a red throat, enlarged cervical lymph nodes, and tiny aphthous ulcers on the tongue. Throat, blood, and urine cultures are negative. Complete blood counts are typically normal. Moderate elevation of the sedimentation rate may be seen during acute episodes. A hallmark is the predictable intervals of the fever; parents often call the pediatrician's office and make an appointment for the following week because they know from prior experience that the child will have the fever at that time.

Diagnosis

PFAPA syndrome may be more common than previously documented. Diagnostic criteria for the PFAPA syndrome have been published and are as follows:

- Recurring fevers beginning before 5 years of age
- Symptoms occurring in the absence of upper respiratory tract infection with at least one of the following signs: aphthous ulcers, pharyngitis, cervical lymph node swelling
- Completely asymptomatic intervals between episodes with normal growth and development
- Exclusion of cyclic neutropenia

Management

Treatment of children with the PFAPA syndrome consists of a single dose of prednisone, 2 mg/kg, which results in a dramatic cessation of fever. This abrupt resolution of fever following prednisone has been proposed as a possible criterion for diagnosis. It has been noted that administration of prednisone may cause febrile episodes to occur more frequently. Tonsillectomy has been reported to eliminate the periodic fever entirely up to 80% of children.

Cyclic Neutropenia

Etiology

Cyclic neutropenia is characterized by recurrent episodes of neutropenia, usually every 21 to 28 days. Recent evidence points to autosomal-dominant genetics in most cases, often associated with a mutation of the gene for neutrophil elastase.

Presentation

Patients usually become symptomatic in childhood. Affected children present with fever, mouth ulcers, and frequently bacterial infections. Fever in children with cyclic neutropenia can also be present in the absence of any identifiable infection. Neutropenia typically can be documented to last 3 to 6 days.

Diagnosis

To make the diagnosis of cyclic neutropenia, serial white blood cell count with differential must be done two or three times per week for 6 weeks. The diagnosis of cyclic neutropenia is made if an absolute neutrophil count greater than $500/m^3$ is seen with subsequent recovery.

Management

Lifelong treatment with granulocyte colony-stimulating factor (G-CSF) has been helpful in many cases.

Hyperimmunoglobulinemia D Syndrome

Etiology

The hyperimmunoglobulinemia D syndrome was first described in the mid-1980s. Most described patients are of Dutch or French heritage. Hyperimmunoglobulinemia D syndrome is thought to be caused by a mutation in the gene encoding mevalonate kinase *(MVK)*. Enzyme activity is diminished although not entirely reduced. It is thought that this mutation somehow causes a decrease in inflammatory cytokines.

Presentation

The syndrome is characterized by recurrent attacks of fever, typically occurring every 4 to 8 weeks. Febrile episodes last about 5 days and can be associated with cervical lymphadenopathy, abdominal pain, and headache.

A hallmark is the high immunoglobulin D (IgD) levels, more than 100 IU/mL or 14 mg/dL. Increased levels of IgA, often in the 1,000- to 2,000-mg/dL range, are also reported.

Diagnosis

Diagnosis is made by evaluation of the clinical history and serum immunoglobulins D levels. Mutation analysis of the *MVK* gene is available at certain reference laboratories.

Management

Treatment is with prednisone at a dose of 1 mg/kg given at onset of fever and repeated 24 hours later. As in the case of PFAPA, this is often thought to abort attacks and cause a decrease in the number of febrile days.

SELECTED READINGS

Berlucchi M, Meini A, Plebani A, et al. Update on treatment of Marshall's Syndrome (PFAPA syndrome): report of five cases and review of the literature. *Ann Otol Rhinol Laryngol* 2003;112 (4):365–369.

Genizi J, Miron D, Spiegel R, et al. Kawasaki disease in very young infants: high prevalence of atypical presentation and coronary arteritis. *Clin Pediatr* 2003;42(3):263–267.

John CC, Gilsdorf JR. Recurrent fever in children. *Pediatr Infect Dis J* 2002;21(11)1071–1077.

Majeed HA. Differential diagnosis of fever of unknown origin in children. *Curr Opin Rheumatol* 2000;12(5):439–444.

Saulsbury FT. Hyperimmunoglobulinemia D and periodic fever syndrome (HIDS) in a child with normal serum IgD but increased serum IgA concentration. *J Pediatr* 2003;143(1):127–129.

Steele RW. Fever of unknown origin: a time of patience with your patients. *Clin Pediatr* 2000;39 (12):719–720.

Steele RW, Jones SM, Lowe BA, et al. Usefulness of scanning procedures for diagnosis of fever of unknown origin in children. *J Pediatr* 1991;119(4):526–530.

Talano JA, Katz BZ. Long term follow-up of children with fever of unknown origin. *Clin Pediatr* 2000; 39(12):715–717.

19

Infection in Solid Organ Transplant Recipients

The past decade has brought a great increase in the number of pediatric patients undergoing solid organ transplantation. Although initially cared for by hospital-based specialists, after transplantation they often receive ongoing care from primary care physicians.

INFECTIONS IN THE FIRST MONTH

Infections in solid organ transplantation are typically grouped according to the time following transplantation. In the first month after transplantation, most infections are related to the actual surgical procedure of transplantation. Patients undergoing transplantation are often colonized with a wide variety of bacterial or fungal pathogens. These pathogens may become invasive after surgery with the resultant placement of catheters and surgical drains. An evaluation for infection in the first weeks after transplantation should focus on the sites of surgical incision and any indwelling catheters. Empiric treatment is difficult because the causative bacteria may be related to the nosocomial pathogens found in a particular hospital setting. Knowledge of these pathogens, including methicillin-resistant *Staphylococcus aureus*, vancomycin-resistant enterococcus, and resistant gram-negative enteric organisms, can help guide empiric therapy.

LATENT INFECTIONS IN TRANSPLANTATION

After the first month of transplantation, infections in the transplant recipient change from nosocomial pathogens to the activation of latent infections. A latent infection is one in which the patient has had past exposure and, although currently asymptomatic, has not completely cleared the pathogen. This is a common occurrence with many of the herpesviruses, including herpes simplex virus, cytomegalovirus (CMV), and Epstein-Barr virus (EBV). The activation of latent infections causing symptomatic or "active" disease is a major cause of morbidity and mortality in the transplant recipient.

It is also important to realize that in the transplant recipient, there are actually two individuals: the donor and the recipient. For a number of latent infections, including EBV, CMV, and toxoplasmosis, the greatest risk for activation occurs when the donor is seropositive (D+) and the recipient is seronegative (R−). This designation of D+/R− is often referred to as a **mismatch**. When a mismatch occurs, the process of transplantation often resembles an acute (primary) infection in the recipient. Primary infection in the setting of intense immunosuppression has a high likelihood of causing symptomatic disease. Documentation of donor and recipient status is very important in evaluating the possibility of infection in a transplant recipient in the months after transplantation.

Additional terms frequently used in describing solid organ transplantation infection include **secondary infection**, in which the previously exposed recipient (R+) has a latent infection reactivate during the course of immunosuppression. **Superinfection** refers to the case in which both donor and recipient are seropositive. Because there is often heterogenicity among various viral strains, the reactivation of the donor strain after transplantation and intense immunosuppression may result in clinical disease. Because of this heterogenicity of viral infections, one cannot assume that a D+/R+ transplantation will have no subsequent problems with that particular latent infection.

Certain latent infections are frequently seen in the transplant recipient. The following is a discussion of these infections and their typical presentation and diagnosis.

CYTOMEGALOVIRUS

Etiology

CMV, a double-stranded DNA virus, is the most important pathogen affecting transplant recipients. Infection can occur at the time of transplantation, often through a D+/R− mismatch. Seronegative recipients of organs from seropositive donors have a greater than 50% risk for the development of symptomatic CMV disease following their primary infection.

Presentation

The manifestations of CMV disease in the transplanted patient include prolonged fever, often with accompanying leukopenia and hepatitis. Pneumonia, colitis, and long-term graft dysfunction are additional manifestations of active CMV disease in the transplant patient.

Diagnosis

Serology is of little value in the diagnosis of CMV disease in transplant patients because even previously seronegative individuals may not reliably produce an adequate antibody response. Several specific techniques are used to diagnose CMV infection. A shell vial assay refers to a technique whereby fibroblast cells are grown in monolayers in a special shell vial container. Clinical specimens are placed within this container and, after 1 to 2 days of incubation, are stained with a monoclonal antibody specific for early CMV antigen. This technique is quicker and more sensitive than conventional viral cultures. In addition, polymerase chain reaction (PCR; nucleic acid amplification) can be used to quantitate CMV in blood or other body fluids. Symptomatic CMV infection is often preceded by viremia. Treatment is sometimes considered in patients who show increasing viral loads by PCR.

Management

The treatment of clinical CMV disease is intravenous ganciclovir at 5 mg/kg given intravenously every 12 hours for a minimum of 2 weeks or until clearance of the viremia is documented. It is important to document the resolution of viremia because the clinical relapse rate in patients with persisting viremia can be greater than 50%. CMV hyperimmune globulin is also available and is often used in the treatment of severe or relapsing disease.

There is increasing appreciation of CMV that is ganciclovir resistant. The overall incidence is about 2%, but certain transplant populations have increased risk. Risk for cytomegaloviral ganciclovir resistance is thought to include mismatch at the time of transplantation, high CMV viral load, kidney-pancreas transplantation, and treatment that results in suboptimal concentrations of ganciclovir. Documentation of ganciclovir resistance in CMV disease involves the identification of a variety of mutations by PCR. This technique is difficult, and in practical terms, ganciclovir resistance is often suspected when patients fail to respond to ganciclovir, as determined by clinical evaluation or by rebound in CMV viral load. Treatment with foscarnet has been used for infection due to ganciclovir-resistant CMV.

Prevention

Because of the high morbidity associated with CMV infection in transplant patients, a variety of strategies have been employed to reduce the risk for symptomatic disease. These strategies are particularly important in patients with the highest risk for developing CMV disease (i.e., patients with D+/R− mismatch and CMV-positive patients undergoing intense immunosuppression). Prophylaxis for CMV refers to the use of ganciclovir postoperatively in selected patients. Patients may receive sequential intravenous and then oral ganciclovir for as long as 100 days after transplantation. CMV-positive individuals receiving antilymphocyte antibody for the treatment of rejection often receive preventive ganciclovir therapy for as long as 3 months to limit viral reactivation. Other centers use "preemptive therapy," which involves the close monitoring of patients with viral load assays or CMV antigenemia assays. Patients who develop viremia, thought to be a predictor of subsequent clinical disease, are then treated with antiviral agents.

Cytomegalovirus

1. Mononucleosis syndrome with fever, leukopenia, hepatitis
2. Colitis
3. Pneumonia
4. Diagnosis
   a. Viral culture
   b. PCR
   c. Bronchoalveolar lavage (viral culture)
   d. Biopsy (showing intra-cellular viral inclusions)

EPSTEIN-BARR VIRUS

Etiology

EBV is the major cause of posttransplantation lymphoproliferative disease (PTLD). PTLD is the term given for a spectrum of EBV-related disorders in the transplant population that range from infectious mononucleosis to monoclonal lymphoma. Primary disease that occurs after transplantation causes the most severe illness. The increase in pediatric transplantations has led to an increased number of transplant recipients who will be getting primary EBV infection after transplantation with resultant increased risk for PTLD.

EBV infection initially targets host B lymphocytes. Cellular immune response is a key element in control of EBV-infected B cells. B-cell proliferation of EBV infection is normally contained by natural killer (NK) cell activity. The inhibition of T-cell immunity by the immunosuppressive regimens given to transplant patients inhibits this protective mechanism and may result in unchecked proliferation of B cells. As B-cell proliferation continues, it is thought to be associated with progressive disease, emerging monoclonality, and progression to lymphoma (Fig. 19.1).

Presentation

There are a variety of clinical manifestations of PTLD, depending on the precise status of the infected B lymphocytes. A severe mononucleosis syndrome with high fever, leukopenia, and hepatitis is often seen. This can be very similar to the clinical picture of symptomatic CMV disease. Enlarging lymphadenopathy may also be a presenting sign. Asymptomatic enlargement of the tonsils may be a sign of PTLD and should always be examined closely in transplant recipients. Intestinal tract involvement, resulting in anorexia, weight loss, and diarrhea, also is a common presentation (Fig. 19.2).

Epstein Barr Infections in Solid Organ Transplant Recipients

Epstein Bar virus Infection (EBV) → B Cells → Polyclonal → Monoclonal → Lymphoma
(Uncontrolled Bcell proliferation)

T cell control of EBV infected B cells decreased by

immunosuppression given to prevent rejection

FIG 19.1. Epstein-Barr virus infections in solid organ transplant recipients.

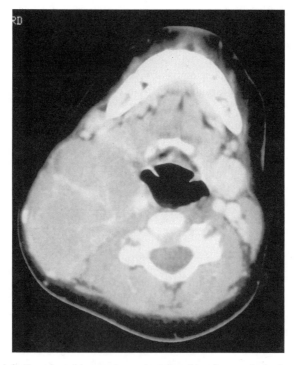

FIG. 19.2. Infections in solid organ transplantation. Massive cervical adenopathy in a patient with posttransplantation lymphoproliferative disease (PTLD).

Diagnosis

The gold standard of diagnosis of PTLD is lymph node biopsy. Biopsy will show the normal lymphoid tissue replaced with a proliferation of B cells in varying stages of transformation. Histologic classification for PTLD is based on the appearance of these B cells. The World Health Organization has suggested the classifications of monomorphic, polymorphic, monoclonal, polyclonal, and Hodgkin's-like PTLD. Progression to malignancy is associated with progressive monoclonality from polymorphic or polyclonal lymphoid hyperplasia.

The measurement of EBV viral load by PCR in peripheral blood or tissue is frequently used in the evaluation of PTLD. These results can be difficult to interpret because differing laboratories use different threshold values as well as different units. A viral load of greater than 4,000 copies/mL of blood is thought to be extremely elevated and in the right clinical context suggests PTLD. Serial measurements of EBV viral loads can be used to follow clinical course; achieving a viral load of less than 200 copies has been correlated with restoration of host immune response and successful resolution of PTLD.

Management

The mainstay of therapy in the treatment of PTLD is reduction or elimination of immunosuppression. This restores T-cell immunity, which then controls the unchecked B-cell proliferation. Heart transplant recipients may need to be monitored in the hospital setting, to receive daily echocardiograms and weekly cardiac biopsy. Antiviral therapy with ganciclovir has been used in treatment of PTLD. Latent B cells represent greater than 90% of the PTLD population, and this population is not amenable to antiviral therapy. Antivirals are often employed in the hope that they may provide some clinical benefit by addressing the remaining 10% of the B-cell population. Rituximab, a monoclonal antibody to the B-cell CD20 antigen, has been used in patients who fail to respond to the elimination of immunosuppression and whose lymphoid biopsy shows this antigen. Chemotherapy has also been used when other treatment modalities have failed or initial presentation is that of monoclonal lymphoma.

Epstein-Barr Virus

1. Posttransplantation lymphoproliferative disease
2. Diagnosis
   a. Serology—generally not helpful
   b. PCR
   c. Biopsy of affected lymph nodes

TOXOPLASMA GONDII

Etiology

Toxoplasma gondii is a common infection. Cats are the primary host; they acquire the infection by eating other animals or undercooked meats. Oocysts are then excreted and can infect another host. Toxoplasmosis is a latent infection that can be transmitted at the time of organ transplantation. Because the myocardium is one of the sites where latent cysts are located, it is more frequent in cardiac transplantation. The greatest risk is in patients who have the D+/R− mismatch.

Presentation

Symptomatic disease usually occurs within the first 6 months after transplantation. Patients may present with organ system involvement, including chorioretinitis, myocarditis, and intracranial lesions.

Diagnosis

Diagnosis is primarily by demonstrating tachyzoites within biopsy specimens; diagnosis can also be suggested by specific toxoplasmosis serology.

Management

Most of the experience in the treatment of toxoplasmosis is derived from the management of patients with acquired immunodeficiency syndrome (AIDS). Pyrimethamine plus sulfadiazine, given in conjunction with folinic acid, is the standard treatment in this population and is often used in infected patients after organ transplantation. Up to 6 weeks of therapy for acute disease is recommended.

Prophylaxis with trimethoprim-sulfamethoxazole (Bactrim) is typically recommended if such a mismatch for toxoplasmosis is documented.

Toxoplasmosis

1. Latent in myocardial tissue
2. Disease manifested as myocarditis, retinitis, brain lesion
3. Diagnosis by biopsy, serology

BK VIRUS

Etiology

BK virus is a human polyomavirus increasingly appreciated as a major cause of morbidity in renal transplantation. BK virus is similar to other viral infections in that seroprevalence in the general population approaches 90%. After acquisition in childhood, the virus establishes latency in renal tubular epithelial cells. Polyomavirus viruria can be found in up to one half of renal transplant recipients in the first 3 months after transplantation.

Presentation

After transplantation and the initiation of immunosuppression, the progressive viral infection may cause ureteral stenosis, hemorrhagic cystitis, and polyomavirus allograft nephropathy (PVAN). The reason for progression of BK renal infection in certain transplant recipients remains unclear; it is speculated that certain risk factors, including graft rejection and HLA mismatch, may play a role. Nearly one half of patients who go on to develop PVAN ultimately lose their graft. The initial manifestation of progressive BK renal infection may be progressive elevation in the serum creatinine and a failure to respond to antirejection or antimicrobial therapy.

Diagnosis

Renal epithelial cells infected with BK virus develop large nuclei and ground-glass intranuclear inclusions termed **decoy cells**. These renal cells are shed in the urine and can often be found by cytologic examination of urine.

The presence of BK viruria can be assessed by urine cytology, enzyme-linked immunosorbent assay (ELISA) antibody detection, or PCR. Interpretation of urine studies may be difficult because such a large number of patients in the immediate posttransplantation period excrete virus in their urine. Persistent urinary shedding of decoy cells associated with BK viremia is often seen in patients who ultimately develop PVAN. Serum PCR is thought to be better at distinguishing those at risk for actual development of nephropathy and is often used as a potential screening test for kidney involvement. Definitive diagnosis of PVAN requires renal biopsy; positive biopsies typically reveal an intense cellular infiltrate associated with viral inclusions.

Management

There is no consensus on the optimal treatment of PVAN. Reduction of immunosuppression is the recommended therapy; the new antiretroviral agent cidofovir has been reported effective in small numbers of patients.

BK Virus

1. Ninety percent seroprevalence in general population
2. High incidence of urinary excretion after transplantation
3. Nephropathy evaluated by serum PCR, renal biopsy

STRONGYLOIDIASIS

Etiology

Strongyloides stercoralis is a common parasite nematode endemic in Southeast Asia, Latin America, and parts of the southeastern United States. In the United States, the highest rates are found in Kentucky and Tennessee. This parasite is remarkable for its ability to persist and replicate in the gastrointestinal tract for many years while producing minimal symptoms.

Presentation

Patients undergoing transplantation, particularly those receiving corticosteroids, are at risk for disseminated disease. Disseminated disease is characterized by overwhelming pulmonary and gastrointestinal involvement, often with concurrent sepsis with gram-negative enteric organisms.

Diagnosis

Patients with disseminated strongyloidiasis often have high eosinophil counts and a distinctive serpiginous skin rash thought to represent intradermal larvae. Definitive diagnosis is made by identification of larvae from stool, bronchoalveolar lavage, or duodenal aspirate.

Management

Treatment is with ivermectin, 200 µg/kg per day for 2 days, although the relapse rate is high in patients with hyperinfection.

Strongyloidiasis

1. Long-term asymptomatic gastrointestinal tract infection
2. Disseminated with eosinophilia, pneumonia, gram-negative sepsis
3. Diagnosis by stool studies, bronchoalveolar lavage, duodenal aspirate

---

FEVER AND PNEUMONITIS IN A TRANSPLANT RECIPIENT

Pneumonia in a transplant recipient is serious and potentially life-threatening. Patients may initially present with a mild increase in respiratory rate with increased work of breathing. Chest x-ray may initially be unremarkable, although hypoxia is frequently seen. Pulmonary infiltrates may appear as the clinical picture proceeds.

The differential diagnosis of fever and pulmonary infiltrates is extensive and includes the following:

- **Bacteria.** Bacterial pneumonia is a particular concern, particularly in patients with concurrent neutropenia. Bacteria such as *Klebsiella pneumoniae* and *Pseudomonas aeruginosa* are common in this setting.
- ***Pneumocystis jiroveci*** (formerly *Pneumocystis carinii*). The reported incidence of *P. jiroveci* pneumonia after transplantation is 2% to 10%. Infection can occur by either reactivation of latent organisms or the acquisition of a new infection. *Pneumocystis* species may cause a diffuse pneumonitis, even when the host is not neutropenic. Patients present with increasing work of breathing and hypoxia; often, the hypoxia occurs before development of pulmonary infiltrates. Continual prophylaxis with trimethoprim-sulfamethoxazole (Bactrim) is often used in transplant patients to reduce the risk for infection. Diagnosis is by bronchoalveolar lavage.
- **"Atypical" pneumonias.** These include the community-acquired pathogens such as *Mycoplasma pneumoniae, Chlamydia pneumoniae,* and *Legionella pneumophila.*
- ***Nocardia* species.** *Nocardia* species may present as progressive pulmonary infiltrates unresponsive to traditional antimicrobial therapy. The radiographic picture is often one of consolidation resembling mycobacterial infection.
- **Viruses.** Viral infection can be a major cause of pneumonia in immunodeficient patients with normal neutrophil counts. Numerous viruses can cause severe pneumonitis and respiratory failure in the transplant recipient; these include respiratory syncytial virus, adenovirus, influenzae virus A and B, parainfluenza virus, CMV, and rhinovirus.
- **Fungi.** Fungal infections that cause pneumonia in transplant patients can be similar to those found in other immunosuppressed patients, including aspergillosis and coccidioidomycosis.
- ***Mycobacterium* species.** These pathogens can include *Mycobacterium tuberculosis* as well as *Mycobacterium avium-intracellulare.*
- **Noninfectious causes.** Not all pulmonary infiltrates are caused by infectious agents. Pulmonary disease in an immunocompromised patient may also be caused by chemotherapy, drug toxicity, and acute respiratory distress syndrome.

The extensive list of possible etiologies of pulmonary infiltrates in a transplant patient makes empiric treatment difficult. Aggressive diagnostic evaluation is required, often by the use of bronchoscopy to obtain bronchoalveolar fluid for specific testing. Testing of bronchoscopy fluid in this setting should include the following:

Bronchoalveolar Lavage Testing

1. Bacterial culture
2. Fungal stain and culture
3. Acid-fast stain and culture
4. *Pneumocystis* species stains
5. Viral culture and specific testing by direct fluorescent antibody to respiratory syncytial virus, adenovirus, influenza, CMV, and herpes simplex virus

---

Empiric treatment often includes a third-generation cephalosporin, an aminoglycoside, trimethoprim-sulfamethoxazole (which will cover both *Pneumocystis* and *Nocardia* species), and often ganciclovir (to cover the possibility of CMV). As diagnostic studies become available, this empiric treatment can be altered as indicated.

SELECTED READINGS

Isada CM, Yen-Lieberman B, Lurain NS, et al. Clinical characteristics of 13 solid organ transplant recipients with ganciclovir resistant cytomegalovirus infection. *Transpl Infect Dis* 2002;4(4):189–194.

Fishman JA, Rubin RH. Infection in organ transplant recipients. *N Engl J Med* 1998;338(24):1741–1751.

Kwak EJ, Vilchez RA, Randhawa P, et al. Pathogenesis and management of polyomavirus infection in transplant recipients. *Clin Infect Dis* 2002;35(9):1081–1087.

Van der Bij W, Speich R. Management of cytomegalovirus infection and disease after solid organ transplantation. *Clin Infect Dis* 2001;33(Suppl 1):S32–S37.

20

Prophylaxis

Prophylaxis refers to the administration of antibiotics not to treat an existing illness but rather to prevent disease from occurring.

Pediatrics is considered a preventative health care specialty, and there is great interest in the specific times when medications are given for the prevention of infection. In general, prophylaxis involves administration of antimicrobials for a brief and specific time period. This chapter discusses some major prophylaxis issues in pediatrics.

RHEUMATIC FEVER

Etiology

Acute rheumatic fever is the result of a preceding *Streptococcus pyogenes* (group A streptococcus) infection. Acute rheumatic fever can occur only after an upper respiratory tract infection. It is thought that postinfection antistreptococcal antibodies generated by the host cross-react with antigens in the brain, heart, and synovial tissue.

Presentation

Because antistreptococcal antibodies can cross-react with any number of organ systems, there are a myriad of presentations of rheumatic fever. It is for this reason that the Jones criteria have been devised for diagnosis.

Diagnosis

The diagnosis of acute rheumatic fever (ARF) is made using the Jones criteria. These criteria are divided into major and minor criteria. The diagnosis of

ARF is made when a patient has two major criteria or one major and two minor criteria.

Jones Criteria: Major Criteria

- **Carditis.** Cardiac involvement in rheumatic fever can affect all areas of the heart, including the myocardium, pericardium, and endocardium. Involvement of the valves is a classic finding in rheumatic heart disease, whereas inflammation of other areas of the heart is more variable. Most cases of valvular disease in rheumatic heart disease involve the mitral or aortic valve. Initial manifestations typically result in valvular insufficiency, with valvular stenosis developing over several decades after initial infection (Fig. 20.1).
- **Arthritis.** The arthritis of rheumatic fever is frequently migratory, with initially affected joints having resolution of arthritis without deformity as subsequent joints become inflamed. A classic finding of the arthritis of rheumatic fever is the dramatic response to aspirin therapy.
- **Chorea.** Patients with chorea have uncontrollable writhing movements, often accompanied by extreme emotional liability and the inability to sit still. The one major exception to the Jones criteria in the diagnosis of ARF is Sydenham's chorea, which occurs in about 15% of patients and alone may make the diagnosis of acute rheumatic fever. Because the onset may be several months after the initial pharyngitis, serologic evidence of the proceeding streptococcal infection may have disappeared.
- **Erythema marginatum.** This is the rash of acute rheumatic fever described as serpiginous macular lesions, primarily on the trunk and extremities.
- **Subcutaneous nodules.** These rare manifestations of acute rheumatic fever are usually associated with severe carditis and are most commonly located on extensor surfaces of tendons.

Jones Criteria: Minor Criteria

- Arthralgia
- Fever
- Laboratory evidence includes elevated acute-phase reactants (sedimentation rate, C-reactive protein) and prolonged P-R intervals on electrocardiogram

---

The diagnosis of acute rheumatic fever also requires evidence of antecedent group A streptococcal infection, which includes a positive throat culture, positive rapid antigen test, or elevated or rising streptococcal antibody titers.

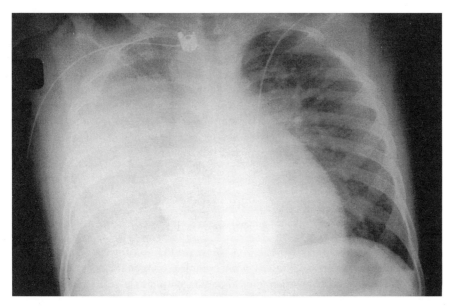

FIG. 20.1. Chest x-ray showing cardiomegaly and pulmonary edema in child with acute rheumatic fever.

The clinical presentation of pediatric acute rheumatic fever may vary with age. Recent reports have stated that children younger than 5 years of age are more likely to present with arthritis and rash and less likely to have chorea. Carditis may be more severe in younger children with resultant chronic cardiac disease.

Management

Prophylaxis of Rheumatic Fever

Prophylaxis of acute rheumatic fever is given in patients after the diagnosis by Jones criteria. The purpose of prophylaxis is to decrease subsequent group A streptococcal infection, which would result in another antibody response with resultant exacerbation of rheumatic disease. There are three chemoprophylaxis regimens of acute rheumatic fever:

1. Benzathine penicillin, 1.2 million units given intramuscularly every 4 weeks
2. Penicillin VK, 250 mg twice a day. For the patient who is allergic to penicillin, erythromycin, 250 mg twice a day, can also be used.
3. Sulfadiazine or sulfisoxazole, 0.5 g once daily for children weighing 60 pounds or less; 1 g for children weighing more than 60 pounds

Duration of Prophylaxis

The duration of prophylaxis for rheumatic fever is often debated. Rheumatic fever with carditis and residual heart disease requires prophylaxis for at least 10 years since the last episode of carditis and at least until 40 years of age. Some experts recommend lifelong prophylaxis to protect an already affected heart. In patients with rheumatic fever with carditis but without residual valvular disease, it is recommended that the duration of prophylaxis is 10 years or into adulthood, whichever is longer. For patients with rheumatic fever without carditis, the duration is 5 years or until 21 years of age, whichever is longer.

ASPLENIA

Etiology

Anatomic or functional asplenia may increase the risk for sudden sepsis with encapsulated organisms. Children with complex congenital heart disease frequently have accompanying asplenia. Patients with sickle cell anemia are considered functionally asplenic secondary to repeated splenic infarctions. *Streptococcus pneumoniae* is the most common infection in these children, although *Haemophilus influenzae*, *Neisseria meningitidis*, and even *Salmonella* species are also seen.

Presentation

Asplenic patients who develop invasive bacterial disease can present initially with fever. There is often rapid progression to septic shock. Petechiae and purpura fulminans, usually seen in meningococcal disease, is not uncommon in asplenic patients with pneumococcal sepsis.

Management

Antibiotic prophylaxis against pneumococcal infections is considered standard of care for all children with asplenia. Oral penicillin V, 125 mg twice daily for children 5 years of age or younger and 250 mg given orally twice a day for children older than 5 years is recommended. In addition to antimicrobial prophylaxis, pneumococcal conjugate and/or polysaccharide vaccines, are indicated. Children with asplenia should also receive the meningococcal polysaccharide vaccine at age 2 years or older. In patients with asplenia, prophylaxis until at least 5 years of age is indicated. Many physicians continue lifelong prophylaxis because the risk for sudden sepsis is decreased but not eliminated. Prophylaxis does not completely eliminate the risk, however, and febrile episodes in patients with asplenia should always be aggressively evaluated and often presumptively treated.

BACTERIAL MENINGITIS

Etiology

One of the most feared infectious diseases in pediatrics is bacterial meningitis (see Chapter 11). There is the concern that the index case may cause subsequent colonization and infection in a close contact. The two organisms that cause bacterial meningitis in which prophylaxis is indicated are *N. meningitis* and *H. influenzae*.

Management

Chemoprophylaxis for families of a child with *N. meningitis* is recommended for children who have had close contact with the index case; this includes household contacts and childcare contacts during the previous 7 days. Individuals who have direct exposure to the patient's secretions, such as a boyfriend or girlfriend or caretakers who have participated in mouth-to-mouth resuscitation or deep suctioning, are also candidates for prophylaxis.

Antibiotic Regimens for Prophylaxis of Meningococcal Disease

- Rifampin, 10 mg/kg (max. 600 mg) in children older than 1 month (given twice a day for 2 days)
- Ceftriaxone, 125 mg given intramuscularly for children 12 years of age and younger; 250 mg given intramuscularly for children older than 12 years
- Ciprofloxacin, 500 mg orally in a single dose for patients older than 18 years

---

In the case of *H. influenzae* type B meningitis, the risk for secondary disease among unimmunized household contacts younger than 4 years of age is the primary concern. Recommendations for chemoprophylaxis are slightly different from those for *N. meningitidis* because it centers on protecting household contacts who have not been fully immunized and thus are vulnerable to invasive disease.

If there is a contact in the home of the index case younger than 4 years of age who is incompletely immunized, all household contacts, including the index case, should receive prophylaxis. One can see that this strategy is focused on protecting the vulnerable patient within the household. If a member of the household is immunocompromised, all occupants receive prophylaxis regardless of the immunization history. Rifampin is not to be given to pregnant women. The prophylaxis regimen is rifampin given once a day in dose of 20 mg/kg up to a maximum of 600 mg. This should be given for 4 days total.

PREVENTION OF PERINATAL GROUP B STREPTOCOCCAL DISEASE

Etiology

Streptococcus agalactiae, or group B streptococcus (GBS), is a major cause of morbidity and mortality in pediatrics. Up to one half of adult women may harbor GBS in their genital tract; antibiotic treatment will not permanently reduce this colonization in adults. At the time of delivery, the bacteria may then colonize the skin of the newborn infant. Although a good percentage of newborns born to colonized mothers themselves become colonized, only a small percentage of these neonates develop invasive disease. Risk factors for invasive GBS disease include premature delivery at less than 37 weeks' gestation, maternal temperature greater than 38°C (100.4°F), and prolonged rupture of membranes greater than 18 hours.

Presentation

GBS disease is divided into two groups: early onset (first week of life) and late onset (up to 3 months of age). Early-onset disease usually presents within the first 24 hours of life with fever, respiratory distress, and sepsis. It is against early-onset disease that prophylaxis regimen is likely to be most effective.

Management

Maternal treatment before delivery has not been found to decrease maternal colonization; therefore, efforts have focused on treatment of the mother at the time of delivery. The theory behind this strategy is that treatment will temporarily decrease colonization in the mother and decrease subsequent colonization and invasive disease in the newborn.

Intensive efforts have been made to determine the best preventative strategy for perinatal GBS disease. Considerable debate exists about whether prophylaxis should be given to all colonized women or just colonized women who exhibited specific risk factors for neonatal invasive disease. In 2002, the Centers for Disease Control and Prevention revised previous recommendations.

New Recommendations for Prevention of Neonatal Group B Streptococcal Disease

All pregnant women should be screened for vaginal and rectal GBS colonization at 35 to 37 weeks' gestation. For women who have positive cultures, intrapartum antibiotics are given. Women who have negative cultures do not require antibiotic prophylaxis, even if there are risk factors for neonatal GBS infection. The recommended regimen is as follows:

Intrapartum prophylaxis for perinatal GBS infection:

- Penicillin G, 5 million units intravenously $\times$1, then 2.5 million units every 4 hours

Alternatives for a maternal history of penicillin allergy:

- Cefazolin, 2 g intravenously $\times$1, then 1 g intravenously every 8 hours
- Clindamycin, 900 mg intravenously every 8 hours
- Erythromycin, 500 mg intravenously every 6 hours

Antibiotic prophylaxis should always use the most narrow spectrum antibiotic possible because there have been reports of increasing *Escherichia coli* resistance to ampicillin, which may be the result of an increasing number of women getting prophylaxis.

Intrapartum prophylaxis is also indicated in the following situations:

1. A mother who had a previous infant with invasive GBS disease
2. GBS bacteriuria during current pregnancy
3. A woman whose GBS status is unknown and has any of the following:
   a. Premature delivery at less than 37 weeks' gestation
   b. Prolonged rupture of membranes greater than 18 hours
   c. Maternal temperature of greater than 38°C (100.4°F)

Mothers who have positive vaginal and rectal cultures during the current pregnancy and have a planned cesarean section without labor or rupture of membranes do not require intrapartum prophylaxis.

CARE OF THE NEWBORN AFTER MATERNAL PROPHYLAXIS

A major issue following maternal prophylaxis is what to do with the newborn. Certainly, an ill-appearing neonate requires a full diagnostic workup and empiric antibiotic therapy. There is ongoing concern about the well-appearing newborn, especially one whose mother has received prophylaxis with antibiotics and thus may have a decrease in the yield of positive blood cultures. Current recommendations suggest that any child born to a mother with suspected chorioamnionitis (i.e., a fever of greater than 39°C [100.4°F] and two or more clinical or laboratory findings suggesting amniotic fluid infection) requires diagnostic evaluation and empiric antibiotic therapy. All newborns who appear clinically ill should have a lumbar puncture performed. A healthy newborn more than 38 weeks' gestation whose mother received more than 4 hours of prophylaxis may be monitored without laboratory evaluation and discharged after 24 to 48 hours.

Well-appearing premature neonates less than 35 weeks' gestation who have had maternal prophylaxis for more than 4 hours may have a limited evaluation, defined as complete blood count and blood cultures, and then be observed for 48 hours. Newborns more than 35 weeks' gestation whose mothers received less than 4 hours of prophylaxis should have a similar limited evaluation and observation.

The revised guidelines do not cover every conceivable situation faced by a pediatrician or neonatologist. Care must often be individualized based on the history of GBS cultures, a prior history of GBS disease, and the clinical and laboratory evaluation of the particular neonate. Nearly all cases of early-onset GBS disease present in the first days of life; children at risk for invasive disease should certainly be observed for at least 48 hours after delivery.

SELECTED READINGS

Madan A, Adams MM, Phillip AG. Frequency and timing of symptoms in infants screen for sepsis: effectiveness of a sepsis-screening pathway. *Clin Pediatr* 2003;42(1):11–18.

Ottolini MC, Lungren K, Mirkinson LJ, et al. Utility of complete blood count and blood culture screening to diagnose neonatal sepsis in the asymptomatic at risk newborn. *Pediatr Infect Dis J* 2003;22(5):430–434.

Schrag S, Gorwitz R, Fultz-Butts K, et al. Prevention of perinatal group B streptococcal disease. Revised Guidelines from CDC. *MMWR Morb Mortal Wkly Rep* 2002;51(RR-11):1–22.

Tani L, Veasy G, LuAnn M, et al. Rheumatic Fever in children younger than 5 years: in presentation different. *Pediatrics* 2003;112(5):1065–1068.

Subject Index